HANDBOO
DENTAL SURGER\
AND OT]
ANCILLARY WORKERS

Handbook for
Dental Surgery Assistants
and other Ancillary Workers

by
Stanley Gelbier
L.D.S. R.C.S.(Eng.), D.D.P.H.

Area Dental Officer,
Lambeth, Southwark and Lewisham Area Health Authority (Teaching);
Examiner for the Diploma in Dental Health Education
(Royal Society of Health)

*Formerly Examiner for the National Certificate for Dental Surgery Assistants
and Lecturer in Child Dental Health at the London Hospital Medical College*

and

Margaret A. H. Copley
S.R.N., S.C.M., D.T.N. & H., Parentcraft Teaching Certificate and
Technical Teacher's Certificate

*Formerly Tutor to National Nursery Examination Board Courses, Middlesex
and to Dental Surgery Assistants, Middlesex,
and Examiner for the National Nursery Examination Board
Member of the Association of British Dental Surgery Assistants*

with a Foreword by
H. M. Pickard
F.D.S. R.C.S.(Eng.), M.R.C.S., L.R.C.P.

Second Edition

BRISTOL: JOHN WRIGHT & SONS LIMITED
1977

CIP Data
Gelbier, Stanley
  Handbook for dental surgery assistants and
  other ancillary workers. - 2nd ed.
  1. Dentistry 2. Dental assistants
  I. Title II. Copley, Margaret Ada Hope
  617.6   RK51

  ISBN 0-7236-0464-9

PRINTED IN GREAT BRITAIN BY BILLING & SONS LIMITED
GUILDFORD, LONDON AND WORCESTER

*To all those who have
striven to raise the standards
of achievement of dental
ancillary workers, especially
the Association of
British Dental Surgery Assistants*

ACKNOWLEDGEMENTS

SPECIAL thanks are due to Professor H. M. Pickard who so kindly wrote the Foreword to this book, and also to Mr. H. A. Butler, Director of Publications of Oral Topics Ltd., who gave us much valuable assistance during the preparation of the manuscript. We are grateful to the following people who so kindly helped and advised us: Miss B. Greenwood, Mrs. T. Killick, Miss J. Lewis, Miss J. McLeish, Miss D. Pollack, Miss M. Jean Smith, Mr. R. M. Gillard, Mr. F. Pearne, and Mr. S. Tinkler. Although they offered us many helpful criticisms, any errors of fact or presentation are our own.

Acknowledgement is due to Amalgamated Dental, London, for their assistance in providing the various illustrations of Ash dental instruments, burs, and forceps shown in Chapter X. We thank the Examining Board for Dental Surgery Assistants for allowing us to reproduce some of their past examination questions. We are fully aware that in writing a text of this nature much information is used that has been gained in the past from lectures, books, and from discussions with colleagues. We therefore offer thanks to all those who have stimulated us in this way.

Many thanks are due to the staff of John Wright and Sons Ltd., who have taken so much trouble during the preparation of this book.

We are indebted to Mrs. A. Silber who painstakingly typed the final copy. Special acknowledgement must be given to Marilyn Gelbier, who allowed her husband the long hours of solitude needed to write this book.

PREFACE TO SECOND EDITION

THE main aims of this book are the same as those expressed in the Preface to the first edition. The latter has been favourably received by those for whom it was written, the dental ancillary workers. In order to make it even more convenient for their use, the chapters have been rearranged. Thus anatomy and physiology appear at the beginning, then the other biological and scientific subjects, and finally the dental ones. The definitions have been regrouped as a Glossary. The opportunity has been taken to include mention of some of the more recent dental materials.

It must be appreciated that our prime objective is to provide a theoretical background upon which the ancillaries can base their practical work. However, no handbook can take the place of practical experience, and no attempt has been made to give detailed advice on those aspects of work which can best be learned by practical demonstration.

London   S. G.
September 1977   M. A. H. C.

PREFACE TO FIRST EDITION

OUR object in writing this book is to provide sufficient background knowledge for all varieties of dental ancillary workers, whether they work in the surgery or not. This therefore includes dental surgery assistants, auxiliaries, health educators, hygienists, receptionists, and technicians. We hope to give them sufficient information to make their work that much more interesting, to enable them to understand what is being done and why, and to allow them to discuss dentistry intelligently with patients and other lay people. It is thus not solely intended to help them get through their examinations, although this in itself would be of great value. Over the years students and teachers have made us increasingly aware of the need for such a book.

London   S.G.
June, 1972   M.A.H.C.

CONTENTS

FOREWORD

By H. M. PICKARD

Emeritus Professor of Conservative Dentistry
Royal Dental Hospital of London

THE dental profession has been slow in appreciating the contribution that can be made by a competent, well-trained, and properly motivated dental surgery assistant. There is some evidence, however, that this phase is passing and that the assistant of the future will be regarded much more realistically as a team member, of whom an ever higher standard of performance is demanded.

In all auxiliary roles it is difficult to know just how much knowledge an assistant should have; in the field of human biology this presents a major problem. In this textbook the authors have assembled a wide range of information, all of it relevant, either as specifically dental or as more general background knowledge. The student in training will find more than she needs; the assistant in practice has a comprehensive source of reference, all closely related to dentistry as it is developing in this and in other countries at the present time.

I have no doubt that this marks a major contribution to the development of dental surgery assisting as a highly-trained, knowledgeable, and indispensable part of our professional activity.

CHAPTER I

INTRODUCTION: THE DENTAL SCENE

DENTISTRY IN THE UNITED KINGDOM

In becoming a member of the dental team, the surgery assistant joins that band of people who have tried to help sufferers from toothache since time immemorial. Such helpers were recorded at least 5000 years before Christ. The Babylonians made use of a strange mixture of medical lore and religious exorcism, calling down in their prayers the wrath of their god Ea on 'The worm that causeth toothache'. Since that time much progress has been made both in the science and art of dentistry, and in the organization of individual practices and community dental services. For convenience a few such advances are chronicled below.

1540 An Act of Parliament united the Guild of Surgeons with the larger Guild of Barber-Surgeons. The latter were allowed to practice no surgery except blood-letting and the drawing of teeth.

1557 The first licence in dentistry was granted, giving permission to draw teeth and make teeth clean. For a long time afterwards most dental operators were itinerant tooth-drawers without training, many of them doing this as a part-time job.

1782 Lectures on dentistry were being given in London.

1858 The first dental hospital and school in London was opened by the Odontological Society of London (now The Royal Dental Hospital of London).

1878 Dentist's Act forbade the use of the term 'dentist' by anyone who was not qualified as a medical practitioner or who was not on the dentist's register. This voluntary register was established and kept by the General Medical Council. It did not prohibit practice by unregistered persons.

1921 Dentist's Act prohibited dentistry to those not on the medical or dental registers. The Dental Board of the United Kingdom was set up to govern the profession, acting in conjunction with the General Medical Council.

1956 Dentist's Act set up the General Dental Council to make the profession self-governing; to be closely allied to medicine but not part of it.

1957   Dentist's Act gave the General Dental Council power to create classes of ancillary workers.

Development of State Dentistry

1. School Children

1907   Education Act allowed education authorities to provide medical inspection of children and to employ school medical and dental officers. In the same year the first English children's dental clinic was opened in Cambridge.

1918   Education Act made provision of dental treatment *obligatory* for elementary school children.

1944   Education Act ensured that authorities provided facilities for dental inspection of all children and made arrangements for securing free treatment through the school dental service or elsewhere.

1953   Education (Miscellaneous Provisions) Act placed a more direct duty on education authorities to provide free dental treatment for all pupils.

1959   School Health Service Regulations instructed every local authority to maintain a school dental service within the framework of the school health service.

2. Pregnant and Nursing Mothers and Pre-school Children

1918   Maternal and Child Welfare Act asked Town and County Councils to provide care for expectant and nursing mothers and pre-school children. They were advised to use the same staff as for school children.

1946   National Health Service Act made it *obligatory* to provide dental care for these groups.

3. Total Population

1911   National Health Insurance Act was designed to provide an insurance scheme for those having an income of less than a certain amount. They were compelled to insure themselves against medical expenses at time of illness. A small number of persons earning *more* than this amount volunteered to join. Some dentistry was provided under this scheme.

1946   National Health Service Act was meant to provide a comprehensive health service for everyone, irrespective of earnings. It was to include dentistry. Any person normally resident in the United Kingdom is entitled to receive from the General Dental Service all the treatment necessary to make him/her dentally fit, i.e., to bring about as reasonable a standard of dental efficiency and oral health as is necessary to safeguard the general health.

N.H.S. DENTAL CARE

The pattern of dentistry today has thus developed from the historical progress detailed above. A free dental priority service thus exists for school children, pre-school children, pregnant and nursing mothers, from both general dental practitioners and from the community dental service. Other patients receive dental care from general dental practitioners and from hospital dentists.

The Hospital Dental Service

This provides for:—

a. Provision of consultant advice and treatment for cases of special difficulty referred to hospitals by general dental and medical practitioners, or for patients admitted to hospital as the result of an accident.

b. Comprehensive dental care of all long-stay hospital in-patients.

c. Dental care of short-stay in-patients when this is required for the relief of pain or other emergency, or as part of, or in support of, their general treatment.

d. Treatment of certain out-patients when medical considerations make it desirable.

General Dental Practice

General dental practitioners providing treatment under the National Health Service are remunerated on an items-of-service basis. Instead of receiving a salary for their services, payment is made according to the amount and type of clinical work done related to a set scale of fees.

The dental surgery assistant or receptionist is usually responsible for keeping all records related to claims for payment. Extreme accuracy is essential Any errors noted by the Dental Estimates Board are treated seriously, and the dentist is held responsible. The Board has the authority to investigate discrepancies, and may arrange for patients to be interviewed and examined. It is essential for the surgery assistant to know and understand the current regulations relating to treatment under the National Health Service if she works in a practice providing this treatment. For example, she must know which items of treatment cannot be provided without the prior approval of the Dental Estimates Board, and whether or not the patient has to contribute towards the cost of this. She must also know how to fill in the relevant official forms.

For all this information she should consult the dental surgeon for whom she works and the *Handbook for National Health Service General Dental Practitioners.*

The Dental Estimates Board is the authority which gives approval for certain cases before their treatment can be commenced, and authorizes payment to the dentist following notification from him that treatment has been completed.

Family Practitioner Committee (F.P.C.)

This is the body responsible in each area for making local arrangements for general medical, dental, pharmaceutical, and ophthalmic services to be provided in accordance with regulations made by the Department of Health and Social Security. It enters a dentist's name on its dental list showing that he is willing to provide general dental services under the National Health Service. This does not prevent him from treating other than National Health Service patients.

Dentists, unlike doctors, do not keep restricted lists of patients. The latter are free to obtain treatment from any dentist on the F.P.C.'s list. It is not essential for the patient to live in the area in which a practice is situated and a dentist is free to accept or refuse anyone as a patient. It is possible for a patient to attend a different dentist for subsequent courses of treatment.

When commencing a course of treatment under the National Health Service patients must sign a form stating that they desire this. They also undertake to submit themselves for examination by a Regional Dental Officer of the Department of Health and Social Security if this should be required. The function of this officer is to ensure that public money is well spent and that patients are properly treated.

The Regional Dental Officer is appointed to advise the Minister, the Dental Estimates Board, F.P.C., and dentists on all professional matters related to the provision of dental treatment.

The F.P.C. pays dentists for treatment carried out on National Health Service patients after notification from the Dental Estimates Board that this has been completed.

Private Practice

One must remember that not all dentistry in the United Kingdom is carried out under the auspices of the National Health Service. Much work is done in true private practice, and it is to this that many surgery assistants will be attracted. Some practices mix private and N.H.S. work.

THE DENTAL TEAM

Since 1956 dentistry has been a self-governing profession. However, dentists cannot, and indeed would not want to, work in isolation. They function best as leaders of a team of ancillary workers, including dental auxiliaries, chairside assistants, health educators, hygienists, receptionists, and technicians.

1. Auxiliaries

They are trained to perform all preventive functions, plus actual dental treatment. At present their work is confined to dentistry for children. They may perform simple fillings and extract deciduous teeth under local anaesthesia. Dental auxiliaries work only:—
 a. Under the direction of a dentist.
 b. To a written prescription.
 c. Within the Public Health Service.

2. Chairside Assistants, Receptionists, and Dental Secretaries

In the smaller type of practice one person would carry out the combined duties of chairside assistant, receptionist, and secretary. Larger practices often employ individual members of staff to carry out these separate functions although their duties can be interchangeable by arrangement. Without these most important and essential workers, modern efficient dentistry would be impossible. They are employed in all spheres of dentistry including general dental practice, school clinics, industrial practice, the Armed Forces, and hospitals. Their function is to release the dentist from routine tasks, enabling him to devote his time to highly skilled operative procedures.

3. Health Educators

In recent years these have become an essential part of the dental scene, often giving lectures to school children, parent–teacher associations, mothers' clubs, etc. They usually have a background of work as dental hygienists, surgery assistants or auxiliaries.

4. Hygienists

These ancillary workers carry out scaling and polishing of teeth, dental health education, and topical application of fluorides and other prophylactic substances. They function almost wholly in a preventive sphere, combating dental caries and periodontal disease.

5. Technicians

These are highly skilled people who make prostheses, crowns, bridges, inlays, orthodontic plates, and other appliances prescribed by the dentist. Without them patients would have to do without advanced restorative procedures.

THE BOOK

The work of the whole ancillary team is thus of immense importance. It is for that reason that this handbook has been written. The chapters are so arranged as to allow first a study of the general biological principles upon which the science of dentistry is based. This will make easier the understanding of later chapters dealing with the actual practice of dental surgery.

CHAPTER II

GENERAL ANATOMY AND PHYSIOLOGY

ALL dental workers should have a basic knowledge of the formation and function of the human body. A simple study of this subject will increase their interest, develop an intelligent approach to the handling of patients, and encourage understanding when dealing with patients' medical histories. A more detailed study of the anatomy and physiology of the head, neck, and teeth is essential, and these are dealt with in subsequent chapters.

SYSTEMS OF THE BODY

1. Skeletal.
2. Muscular.
3. Nervous.
4. Respiratory.
5. Circulatory.
6. Lymphatic.
7. Digestive.
8. Endocrine.
9. Urogenital.

These consist of organs formed from tissues, the basic structure of which is the 'cell'. No one system functions independently. All work together to keep the body in good health, the nervous and endocrine systems governing and controlling the others. Following injury or disease compensation may take place due to this teamwork within the body.

Oxygen is essential to life. Should the brain be deprived of this, cell damage or even death will result. A healthy blood-supply within the circulatory system carries a plentiful supply of oxygen plus all other nutrients required for tissue maintenance. Unwanted waste products are carried away via the blood and lymphatic systems.

THE CELL (*Fig.* 1)

The simplest form of life. Living cells are formed from protoplasm ('the physical basis of all life'). This is slightly opaque, colourless, and jelly-like. It contains much water, organic and inorganic salts, glucose, fats, and nitrogenous matter. Its complex make-up may be observed through a microscope.

Every cell is a living unit of the whole body, each with a special structure and active life of its own. The activity of living cells is continuous. During growth and maturation they follow the pattern of

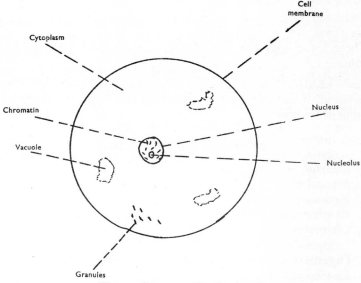

Fig. 1.—Structure of a simple cell.

all living organisms by breathing, excreting, moving, responding to stimuli, producing heat and energy, and reproducing. Cells require oxygen and nutrients for their existence, these being obtained from tissue fluids in surrounding spaces. This fluid passes from the blood, via fine capillary walls, into the tissue spaces. As well as supplying cells with their needs, the fluid also carries away the waste products.

Cell reproduction depends upon the vital centre or nucleus. This consists of thread-like chromatin which contains genes to pass on hereditary characteristics such as hair-colour and height.

Fertilization is the fusion of male (spermatozoa) and female (ovum, or egg) cells. They fuse together to form a zygote, which grows, multiplies, and develops to reproduce further cells.

TISSUES

The earliest formation of human tissue is from the germ-cell lining the fertilized ovum of the female (the blastoderm). It gives rise to *three basic embryonic layers* from which the whole body develops: endoderm, mesoderm, and ectoderm.

Endoderm: Forms lining of the alimentary tract and its glands, except for salivary glands. It also provides most of the lining to the respiratory system.

Mesoderm: Provides connective tissue, muscle, blood and its vessels, lymphatics, bone, dentine, and pulp.

Ectoderm: Produces epithelial layers of skin, hair, nails, oral mucosa, tooth enamel, and nervous tissue.

These layers give rise to *four basic tissues*, which form the body as a whole:—

1. *Epithelium* (*simple and compound*)*:* Lines the circulatory, lymphatic, respiratory, alimentary, and reproductive systems, and forms the outer layer of skin.

2. *Connective Supporting Tissue:* Gives support to other tissues, and is found under the skin, between muscles, inside organs to bind their main structures, forms layers of fat for support and protection, and forms cartilage, bone, and blood.

3. *Muscle:* Voluntary, involuntary, and cardiac.

4. *Nervous tissue:* Forms brain and spinal cord.

SKELETAL SYSTEM

The skeleton gives support and movement to the body as a whole. It consists of 208 bones, varying in size and shape (long, short, flat, irregular, and sesamoid).

It is divided into two main sections: (1) axial, (2) appendicular.

Axial Skeleton

Contains bones of the upright parts of the body, i.e., skull, vertebral column, ribs and sternum.

	No. of bones
Skull	22
Vertebral column	33
Ribs	24
Sternum	1
Total	80

Appendicular Skeleton

Contains shoulder and pelvic girdles, and upper and lower limbs.

	No. of bones
Shoulder girdles and upper limbs	10
Pelvic girdle and lower limbs	10
Hands and wrists	54
Feet and ankles	52
Knees (1 sesamoid bone in each leg)	2
Total	128

Definitions

Joints (Fig. 2): Places where two bones meet.
Sutures: Immovable joints between bones.
Condyle: Smooth rounded projection of bone which forms part of a
mobile joint.

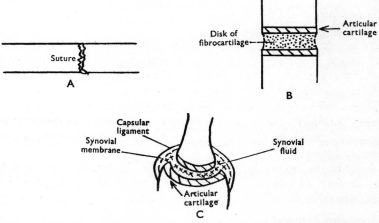

Fig. 2.—Three types of joint. **A,** Simple suture—immovable. **B,** Cartilaginous joint—limited movement possible. **C,** Synovial joint.

Composition of Bone

A hard connective tissue consisting of:—
Water (25 per cent);
Organic material (30 per cent);
Inorganic salts (45 per cent).

Types of Bone

1. *Compact:* Solid outer layer.
2. *Cancellous:* Sponge-like inner layer.

Structure of Bone

Cancellous bone contains red bone-marrow, where red and white blood-cells form and mature, prior to passing into the circulation.

Periosteum is the protective outer covering to bone. It supplies osteoblasts (bone-forming cells) from its deeper layers. Blood-vessels pass through it to supply food and oxygen to the underlying bone.

Development of Bone

For healthy development of bone, mineral salts and vitamins are essential dietary constituents for infants and young children. Calcium, phosphorus, and vitamins A and D must be included in the daily intake.

Many bones develop from cartilage, during foetal growth. Others develop from membranes, and some sesamoid bones develop from tendons.

Two types of bone cells take part in the structure and growth of bone:—

Osteoblasts build bone.

Osteoclasts destroy bone.

There is a constant state of interaction between these two types of cell, bone building and repair being a continuous process throughout life. Osteoclasts produce hollow cavities within the long bones, forming medullary canals for the deposit of bone-marrow.

During the eighth week of foetal growth, cartilaginous long bones develop 'primary centres of ossification' from which developing bone grows, utilizing mineral salts for the purpose. Osteoblasts are very active in this process.

After birth, 'secondary centres of ossification' appear at the ends of bone shafts. The bone then has two areas from which growth and hardening take place, and this process continues until the age of 25.

Functions of Bone

1. To give support and form a framework to the body.
2. To protect vital organs, including brain, heart, and lungs.
3. To provide movement by forming levers.
4. For attachment of muscles.
5. Storage of minerals such as calcium and phosphorus.
6. Formation of blood-cells in the red bone-marrow.

MUSCULAR SYSTEM

Muscles are divided into groups according to their function.

1. Voluntary.
2. Involuntary.
3. Cardiac.

Voluntary (Skeletal or Striped)

Cells are elongated to form fibres. Most of these muscles are attached to bone or skin by muscle-tendon, a fibrous tissue. Because of these attachments the skeleton is supported and able to move. Such muscles are controlled by 'the will'.

Involuntary (Smooth and Plain in Structure)

Found in internal organs, blood-vessels, lymphatics, respiratory, and alimentary systems. They are not controlled by 'the will'.

Cardiac

Found only in the structure of the heart. They are not controlled by 'the will'. Their fibres have a special formation to give strength and movement to the heart.

All muscles are arranged in groups, these working in opposition to each other. As one contracts and pulls, the other relaxes and stretches, producing steady and controlled movements. The whole body is held in an upright position by constant tension of the muscles. Visceral (involuntary) muscles form layers arranged in opposition to each other, giving strength and flexibility.

Muscle Tone

Even when not in actual use, muscles remain in a state of partial contraction, and thus quickly respond to any stimulus. This is known as 'muscle tone'.

Muscle Fatigue

Stimulation normally causes a muscle to contract. If excessive stimuli are received, the muscle becomes fatigued and no longer responds.

Composition of Muscle Tissue

Water (75 per cent);
Protein (20 per cent);
Minerals, glycogen, glucose, and fat (5 per cent).

NERVOUS SYSTEM

Consists of two main parts:—
1. Central nervous system.
2. Autonomic nervous system.

Central Nervous System

A mass of nerve-cells and their processes form the brain, spinal cord, and peripheral nerves. The brain lies within the cranial cavity of the skull, and consists of five parts (*Fig.* 3):—

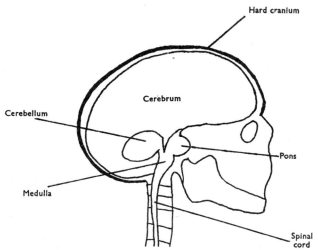

Fig. 3.—Main parts of the brain within its protective cranial box.

1. *Cerebrum* (large brain) formed by a right and left hemisphere. Its nerve-cells form the 'grey matter' of the brain.
2. *Midbrain* (not indicated in *Fig.* 3).
3. *Pons varolii.*
4. *Medulla oblongata.*

The last three of these together form the brain-stem. This is responsible for the passage of nerve stimuli to and from the brain. The medulla oblongata contains vital centres that control cardiac and respiratory systems, as well as the reflex centres for vomiting, coughing, and sneezing. It also influences the walls of blood-vessels, blood-pressure, and body temperature.

5. *Cerebellum* (smaller brain): oval shaped, lying behind the pons varolii. It controls muscular movement, balance, and maintenance of muscular tone, and acts as a co-ordinator between groups of muscles to produce smooth, even, body movements. Thus any damage to this part results in uncoordinated muscle movements, and the gait and balance of the body is affected.

The brain and spinal cord are protected by meninges, three layers of membrane tissue. Within this covering cerebrospinal fluid protects, supports, and maintains an even pressure around the brain and spinal cord. It acts as a shock absorber and keeps the tissues moist.

The spinal cord is about 18 inches long and as thick as a small finger. It lies in the nerve-canal of the vertebral column, and is the nerve link between brain and body organs. Messages reach the brain via the spinal cord, are recorded, interpreted, and then relayed for action to the various organs of the body. Thirty-one pairs of nerves originate from the cord, taking their names from the region in which they pass out of the canal.

Nerves	No. of pairs
Cervical	8
Thoracic	12
Lumbar	5
Sacral	5
Coccygeal	1

Autonomic Nervous System

Controls parts of the body which function automatically without conscious control, e.g., heart-rate, glandular secretion (saliva and sweat), diameter of blood-vessels, relaxation and contraction of muscles, peristalsis of the alimentary tract. Organs are controlled by a balancing interaction between sympathetic and parasympathetic nerves.

EXAMPLES OF SYMPATHETIC REACTIONS

Increased heart-rate and dilatation of arteries brings more blood to organs, the spleen contracts to pour more blood into the circulation, bronchi dilate to allow faster respiration, increased sweat gland activity in the skin allows greater heat loss from this part, thus cooling the body. This combined reaction is known as the 'flight and fight' response, aiding the body to cope with emergencies. Parasympathetic nerves cause the reverse to happen.

Cranial Nerves

Twelve pairs arise directly from the brain. Some are sensory, others motor, and a third group are mixed.

Sensory Nerves: Pass stimuli (e.g., pain, heat, touch) to the brain.

Motor Nerves: Pass messages from brain to muscles and organs, causing them to function, in response to the original stimulus which went to the brain.

Mixed Nerves: Sensory and motor, carrying both types of stimuli.

The twelve pairs of cranial nerves are:—

1. Olfactory: Smell.
2. Optic: Sight.
3. Oculomotor: Eye muscles.
4. Trochlear: Eye muscles.
5. Trigeminal: Sensations from skin of face and forehead, mouth, teeth; motor to muscles of mastication.
6. Abducent: Eye muscles.
7. Facial: Muscles of facial expression; sensation of taste.
8. Auditory: Hearing.
9. Glossopharyngeal: Tongue, tonsils, pharynx, parotid gland secretions.
10. Vagus: Pharynx, larynx, trachea, heart, oesophagus, stomach, small intestine, pancreas, spleen, ascending colon, kidneys, blood-vessels of thorax and abdomen.
11. Accessory: Pharynx, larynx, soft palate, sternomastoid muscle.
12. Hypoglossal: Muscles of tongue.

The trigeminal and facial nerves are intimately concerned with the physiology of the teeth and jaws, and are fully discussed in Chapter III.

RESPIRATORY SYSTEM

Respiration is the mechanism of taking oxygen into the body and eliminating carbon dioxide from it. These gases pass along the air-passages, which consist of the nose, pharynx, larynx, trachea, bronchi, and bronchioles (*Fig.* 4).

The Nose

Divided into two sections by a nasal septum. The central portion is lined with cilia (hair-like structures) which collect dirt, dust, mucus, and other foreign materials. These are then sneezed or blown from the nose, thus protecting the air-passages. Air passing through the nasal passages is warmed by the extensive number of small blood-vessels in their mucous membrane lining.

The Pharynx

Lies behind the nose and mouth. It transmits air into the larynx, and food into the oesophagus. Respiration stops when swallowing occurs.

The Larynx (Adam's Apple)

Lies at the top of the trachea or wind-pipe. It contains the vocal cords and is the organ of voice production.

The Trachea

A tube about four inches in length extending from the larynx to the upper part of the chest, where it divides into right and left bronchi.

The Lungs

Each bronchus enters a lung, where it divides and subdivides like the branches of a tree. The fine tubes (bronchioles) terminate in minute air sacs (alveoli). These are surrounded by a vast network of tiny (thin-walled) capillaries, so that oxygen can easily pass into the bloodstream, and carbon dioxide out of it. The vessels are so narrow that red blood-cells can only pass through in single file, making it easier for gases to pass into, and out of, these cells.

Thus oxygen enters the lungs, is transferred to the pulmonary blood circulation, and then travels via the pulmonary *veins* to the heart. Carbon dioxide and other waste products travel in de-oxygenated blood from the lungs via pulmonary *arteries.*

The right lung is larger than the left one, giving up some space in the chest cavity (mediastinum) for the heart, which lies between the two lungs. The broad parts of the lungs are concave, and lie just above the diaphragm. The apex extends about one inch behind the level of the clavicle (collar-bone).

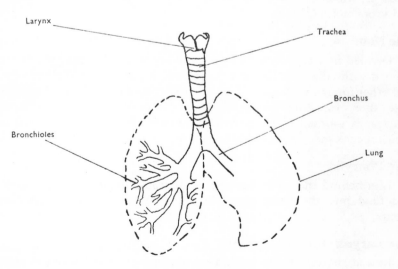

Fig. 4.—The respiratory system.

Mechanics of Respiration

The lungs lie within the rib cage of the chest cavity. Intercostal muscles between the ribs move the cage. Breathing consists of (1) inspiration, (2) pause, and (3) expiration.

Inspiration: Rib cage moves upwards and outwards, and the diaphragm downwards, creating a vacuum around the lungs. This makes them expand, and suck in air.

Expiration: The reverse process. Thus normal breathing has a thoracic and a diaphragmatic component.

Coughing: Forced expiration of air through the narrow opening of the vocal cords.

Sighing and yawning: Prolonged inspiration and expiration.

Hiccough (hiccup): Noisy inspiration due to irregular but sudden movements of the diaphragm.

Tidal air: Air passing in and out of lungs during normal breathing.

Complemental air: Additional air passing during stronger breathing.

Supplemental air: Air expelled from the lungs with force.

Residual air: That remaining in the lungs after normal expiration.

Vital capacity: Volume of air expelled by a deep expiration following a deep inspiration.

Hyperpnoea: Increased depth of respiratory movements.

Apnoea: Temporary stoppage of breathing.

Dyspnoea: Difficult breathing.

Normal adult rate of respiration: 16 to 18 breaths a minute. N.B. An infant may breathe at 40 per minute.

Certain respiratory diseases and other illnesses, drugs, shock, and internal haemorrhage can alter the rate of respiration. Changes in the chemical composition of the blood and nervous impulses may influence respiration, e.g., raising the carbon dioxide level of the blood stimulates the respiratory centre to increase the rate of breathing.

Functions of Lungs

1. Site of gaseous interchange between external environment and blood.

2. Supply of air to the larynx for voice production.

3. Excretion of water vapour.

Atmospheric air contains much oxygen, nitrogen, and a little carbon dioxide.

Expired air contains much carbon dioxide, a little oxygen, and nitrogen. It is warmer and contains water vapour, possibly plus microorganisms as 'droplet infection'.

CIRCULATION OF BLOOD

Blood is transported around the body in an unbroken circuit of vessels. The central point is the constantly beating heart, at a rate of 72 beats per minute (*Fig.* 5).

The Organs of Circulation

1. The heart acting as a pump.
2. Arteries and arterioles transporting pure (oxygenated) blood.
3. Veins and venules transporting impure (de-oxygenated) blood.
4. Networks of capillaries. These extremely thin structures are one cell thick, enabling gaseous exchanges to take place between the circulation and tissue cells.

The Heart

A hollow, muscular, cone-shaped organ lying between the lungs, within the chest cavity or thorax. The apex (tip) rests upon the diaphragm and points towards the left lung, for about $3\frac{1}{2}$ inches. Its broader base lies to the right and above the collar-bone. The sternum passes down in front of it.

THREE LAYERS OF HEART

1. *Pericardium:* Outer fibrous sac consisting of two fine layers of tissue separated by sticky fluid. The latter prevents friction when the heart beats.
2. *Myocardium:* Middle layer forming bulk of organ. It consists of plain and striped muscle-fibres arranged to give maximum strength to force blood out of the heart, and around the circulation.
3. *Endocardium:* Inner lining of membranous tissue. This extends to form the lining of adjoining arteries and veins, and the cusps of the heart-valves which control the flow of blood through the heart chambers.

STRUCTURE OF THE HEART (*Fig.* 6)

The hollow heart-chambers each hold about 4 ounces of blood.
Auricles (*atria*): The two upper chambers.
Ventricles: The two lower chambers.
Before birth the two auricles are connected by an opening (foramen ovale) which allows blood to pass directly from the right to the left side. In addition, a foetal vessel (ductus arteriosus) connects pulmonary artery and aorta, short-circuiting the blood to by-pass the lungs. Shortly after birth, ductus and foramen are obliterated. Sometimes the latter does not close in the normal way, the baby being left with a 'hole in the heart'. This can be repaired by means of surgery.

The nervous mechanism supplying the heart-muscle has one point of communication along the septum or midline—the atrioventricular bundle of His. Thus stimuli produce a corresponding rhythmic beating of the two upper chambers together, followed by the two lower chambers in unison.

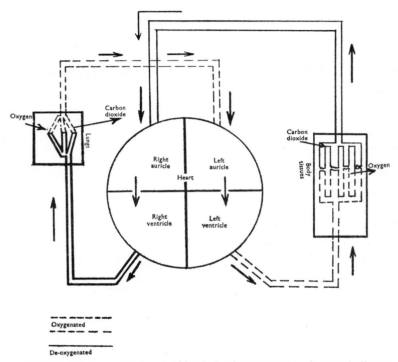

Fig. 5.—Diagram showing the blood circulatory system. Arrows indicate direction of blood flow. Oxygenated blood is carried in vessels indicated by dotted lines. De-oxygenated blood in vessels indicated by unbroken lines.

There is a variation in the thickness of the chamber walls. As ventricles need great pressure to pump blood around the whole body, they have thicker walls than do auricles.

The walls of the auricles are smooth, with a number of muscular projections (papillary muscles) which form fine tendons (chordae tendinae) at their free ends. These extend to the lower borders of the dividing valves between upper and lower chambers. They prevent the valve cusps from being forced up into the atria when the ventricles contract, and thus stop blood from flowing backwards.

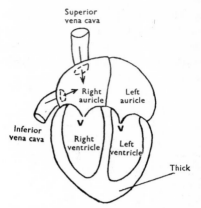

Fig. 6.—Diagram showing structure of the heart; v, valves.

HEART AND VESSEL VALVES

Heart valves consist of tough cartilage, and control the openings between upper and lower chambers:—

1. *Mitral* (*two-cusp*) *valve:* Between left auricle and ventricle.
2. *Tricuspid* (*three-cusp*) *valve:* Between right auricle and ventricle.

The large vessels receiving blood from the heart also have hinge-like valves.

1. *Aortic valve:* Between aortic artery and left ventricle. It consists of three projections from the wall of the vessel. When the ventricle contracts, blood is forced past these cusps. With contraction of the aorta, blood forces the cusps to close, and itself travels along the aorta.
2. *Pulmonary valve:* Similar function for the pulmonary artery on the right side.

THE CORONARY CIRCULATION

Heart-muscle has its own special circulation. This arises in the aorta to form right and left coronary arteries. These supply heart-muscle with fresh oxygenated blood, keeping it in a healthy condition. Drainage from this circulation is direct to the right atrium, where the blood mixes with that entering from the vena cava. Should any of the blood-vessels of this fine circulation be injured or damaged, the heart is affected and may cease to function.

Circulation of Blood through the Heart, Lungs, and Rest of the Body (*Fig.* 7)

1. The right auricle receives venous blood from the upper and lower parts of the body via two vena cavae. The superior vena cava collects

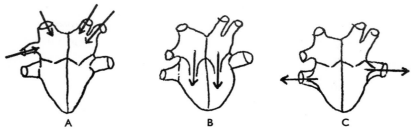

A   B   C

Fig. 7.—Showing way in which blood flows through the heart in one direction, under the control of valves. A, Auricles relaxed, blood flows in from venae cavae and pulmonary veins. B, Auricles contract, blood forced through valves to ventricles. C, Ventricles contract, valves pressed closed, blood forced into aorta and pulmonary arteries.

de-oxygenated blood from the neck, head, and upper limbs. The inferior vena cava drains the lower parts of the body.

2. From the right auricle blood is pumped through the tricuspid valve into the right ventricle. From here it passes into the pulmonary *artery*, which is the only one in the entire body carrying impure blood. It forms two branches, one to each lung.

3. In the lungs blood is circulated through arterioles into a vast network of capillaries. These surround tiny air sacs where gaseous exchange takes place. Pure oxygen is exchanged for impure carbon dioxide. The capillaries have very thin walls and a narrow lumen. Single files of red blood-cells slowly pass through these vessels, giving off their oxygen and taking up the carbon dioxide.

4. The capillaries gradually form venules, from which arise the four main pulmonary *veins*, two from each lung. These carry pure oxygenated blood to the left auricle, thus differing from all other veins in the body.

N.B. The pulmonary arteries and veins together form the pulmonary circulation.

5. From the left auricle blood is pumped through the mitral valve into the left ventricle.

6. From the left ventricle it travels via the aortic valve, to commence its journey around the body.

7. The aorta branches to form a network of arteries supplying all systems of the body with oxygenated blood. As this giant vessel leaves the heart it arches over and above the base of the heart. From there it sends branches to the neck, head, and upper limbs. As it bends downwards it provides branches to the thorax, coronary circulation, liver, stomach, spleen, kidneys, mesentery, groin, organs of reproduction, and the lower limbs.

The Blood

Ninety per cent of the total volume of about 10 pints is water. Blood consists of cells (45 per cent) and plasma (55 per cent).

FUNCTIONS OF BLOOD

1. *Respiration:* Carriage of oxygen from the air and carbon dioxide from the tissues.

2. *Nutrition:* Transport of food material from alimentary canal to tissues.

3. *Excretion:* Removal of waste products of metabolism.

4. *Maintenance of water content of the tissues:* There is a constant interchange of water between blood and tissue fluids.

5. *Regulation of body temperature:* When the body is very warm more blood-vessels open up in the skin, bringing extra blood to the skin surface. Here it loses much of its heat, thus cooling the body.

6. *Carriage of regulative and protective substances:* This includes antitoxins, antibodies, and hormones.

TYPES OF CORPUSCLES OR CELLS

1. *Red (erythrocytes):* 5 million per c.mm. of blood. Contain haemoglobin, which helps to absorb oxygen. Lack of cells or haemoglobin leads to anaemia.

2. *White (leucocytes):* 7000 per c.mm. Act as part of the body defences against invading micro-organisms. They surround and devour bacteria. During the battle leucocytes are also destroyed. These plus dead bacteria and dead tissues in the area form 'pus'. Other white cells gather up the waste and destroy it, the whole process being called 'leucocytosis'.

3. *Platelets (thrombocytes):* 250,000 per c.mm. Take part in the blood-cutting process.

COMPOSITION OF PLASMA

Water (90 per cent);

Proteins; albumin, globulin, fibrinogen;

Mineral salts;

Organic substances, such as glucose, cholesterol, and urea;

Respiratory gases; oxygen, carbon dioxide;

Hormones: chemical agents carried around the body to control various organs;

Enzymes: speed up chemical changes within the body systems;

Antibodies and antitoxins: destroy micro-organisms and their poisons, thus combating infection;

Heparin: an anti-clotting agent.

INCREASE IN NUMBER OF CELLS

Red ones increase during exercise, on top of high mountains, and at high environmental temperatures, thus increasing the oxygen-carrying capacity of blood.

White ones increase as a response to infection.

THE CLOTTING PROCESS

To prevent excessive bleeding (haemorrhage) from damaged blood-vessels, certain chemical processes are set in motion. Damaged tissue cells release a substance called 'thromboplastin'. Together with calcium this produces prothrombin, which is itself converted to thrombin. The latter acts upon fibrinogen (a plasma protein) to produce fibrin. This is a thread-like substance which entangles red and white cells to form a clot. The clot shrinks, and a sticky substance called ' serum ' is released. The process can be summed up as follows:—

$$
\begin{array}{c}
\text{Thromboplastin} + \text{calcium} \longrightarrow \text{prothrombin} \\
\downarrow \\
\text{Fibrinogen} + \text{thrombin} \longrightarrow \text{fibrin} \\
\text{(thread-like)} \\
\text{Traps cells} \downarrow \\
\text{Clot}
\end{array}
$$

THE LYMPH SYSTEM

Fluid from tissue spaces drains into lymphatics (fine capillary-like vessels), circulates around the body, and drains from larger lymph-ducts into veins. Small round glands (nodes) lying alongside some of the vessels act as filters, through which all lymph passes. As bacteria and other foreign bodies cannot pass through, they are filtered off. Lymphocytes are manufactured in nodes; they devour bacteria and foreign bodies, and try to excrete them from the body. With infection the nodes swell and become inflamed, due to the presence of large numbers of bacteria and their toxins.

Oedema

An increased quantity of fluid in a part. This may be due to local trauma or infection, or to a more generalized (systemic) cause. For example, it may be a symptom of heart or kidney disease. It occurs in people who are allergic to shell-fish, strawberries, or penicillin, when the condition is called ' urticaria '. In advanced stages the skin is puffy and, if pressed with a finger, leaves a dent (pitting oedema).

DIGESTIVE SYSTEM AND ALIMENTARY TRACT (*Fig.* 8)

Responsible for ingestion, digestion, assimilation, and absorption of all food and drink. The organs involved are alimentary canal, salivary glands, liver, gall-bladder, and pancreas. The canal consists of mouth, pharynx, oesophagus, stomach, and intestines.

The mouth is sensitive to texture and temperature. Taste-buds on the tongue detect flavours such as salt, sour, sweet, bitter. Teeth start to tear, bite, and chew food, whilst salivary glands pour out their juices. The softened food is ground by the teeth, moved around by the tongue and cheeks to form a bolus, and pushed to the back of the mouth. It is thus guided to the pharynx and oesophagus by muscular action. The cartilaginous epiglottis flaps over the larynx to stop food going into the air-passage instead of that for food.

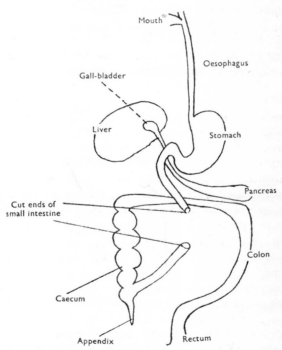

Fig. 8.—Parts of the alimentary system.

The Oesophagus

A muscular tube about 9 inches in length. It passes down, through the diaphragm, to open into the stomach. The bolus travels down by a wavelike peristaltic movement, until it reaches the sphincter muscle guarding the entrance to the stomach. No digestion takes place during this passage.

The Stomach

The entrance to the stomach is guarded by a strong sphincter muscle, which is opened by pressure on either side. It prevents the stomach from filling too quickly. Retching and vomiting may occur if the nerve-supply to the stomach is disturbed.

The stomach lies in the upper left part of the abdomen. It is J-shaped, with the hook passing to the midline, close to the underside of the liver.

It has three strong muscular coats (longitudinal, circular, oblique). An outer moist coat (peritoneum) prevents any friction and covers the other abdominal organs, keeping them in position. The inner lining contains blood-vessels and glands. Gastric juices from these glands break down food to simple chemical components. This lining forms numerous folds. Softened food stays in the stomach for several hours, being churned to ensure full contact with the gastric juices. These are secreted in response to food entering the stomach.

GASTRIC JUICES

1. *Pepsin:* Splits food proteins (body-building foods).
2. *Rennin:* Curdles milk, and is especially abundant in infants.
3. *Lipase:* Splits fats in preparation for further digestion in the small intestine.
4. *Hydrochloric acid:* Provides correct acid environment for other enzymes to act, and destroys bacteria, preventing them from passing into the intestines. Ptyalin from the mouth is neutralized to stop its action. Iron from food is liberated by hydrochloric acid, making it available for uptake into red blood-cells.
5. *Anti-anaemic factor:* Acts upon vitamin B. It is essential for the proper formation of red blood-cells.
6. *Mucin:* Acts as a binding agent.

The exit from the stomach is guarded by the pyloric sphincter. Pressure from food remnants in the stomach causes it to open, allowing the food to pass into the small intestine. Sometimes this sphincter does not easily open, and the food in the stomach creates a great deal of pressure as it cannot get out. This condition of pyloric stenosis sometimes occurs in infants. The child takes some of its food, but this is eventually expelled backwards with great force ('projectile vomiting'). With advancing age the sphincter may harden, also preventing food from easily passing through.

THE SMALL INTESTINE

Food from the stomach enters via the pyloric sphincter. It enters first the duodenum, and then the jejunum and ilium. These three parts measure about 30 inches in length. The constant peristalsis (wavelike movements) mixes food remnants with juices from nearby organs.

The C-shaped duodenum is fixed to the abdominal wall by peritoneum. The bile-duct (from the gall-bladder) and pancreatic duct (from the pancreas) open into it about half-way along its length.

The small intestine has four coats: peritoneal, muscular, submucous, mucous. The last two lie in folds to give a larger internal surface area, aiding secretion and absorption.

The major processes of assimilation and absorption take place in the small intestine. Fats are broken down to glycerol and fatty acids. Carbohydrates are converted to simple sugars such as glucose, maltose, fructose, and sucrose. Proteins finally become simple amino-acids. Glycerol and fatty acids are absorbed via lymphatic tissue in the folds of the mucous membrane.

THE LARGE INTESTINE

About 5 feet long, and divided into caecum and vermiform appendix, ascending colon, transverse colon, descending colon, pelvic colon, and rectum with anal sphincter muscle.

The main functions are:—

1. Lubrication of waste matter, to allow easy passage to anus.

2. Bacteria normally resident in the bowel act upon food residue which has not already been digested or absorbed in the small intestine.

3. The walls of the colon absorb water, glucose, and salt, which are eventually returned to the blood.

The waste remnants (faeces) remain in the lower bowel until pressure from bulk causes opening of the sphincter and defaecation.

Food and Nutrition

Foods of all kinds must be eaten to sustain the body. In addition, oxygen is necessary to burn up (oxidize) these foods, enabling them to then be used in the best way possible. This process is called 'metabolism', which results in the release of energy and heat.

TYPES OF FOODS (NUTRIENTS)

1. *Carbohydrates:* Provide the body with energy, and may be converted to fat, i.e., all starches and sugars.

2. *Fats:* Provide energy and form body fat.

3. *Proteins:* The material for growth and repair of body tissues.

They also provide energy. Animal and vegetable proteins are found in meat, offal, fish, eggs, milk, cheese, and peanuts.

4. *Minerals:* Material for growth and repair, and for regulation of body processes, e.g., calcium, phosphorus, sodium, iodine, and iron. The first two are essential for the formation of strong bones and teeth.

Mineral	Source
Calcium	Milk, cheese, bread, flour, green vegetables
Phosphorus	Cheese, oatmeal, liver, kidney, eggs
Iron	Liver, beef, wholemeal bread

5. *Vitamins:* Regulate the body processes. Available from a wide variety of sources (*Table I*). Lack of vitamins cause deficiency diseases, e.g., Beri-beri (lack of B_1), pellagra (nicotinic acid—part of B-complex), polyneuritis (B_{12}), scurvy (C), and rickets (D).

Vitamins A, D, E, and K are fat-soluble, and may therefore be stored in fat depots in the body. Excessive vitamin D can be dangerous.

Vitamins B and C are water-soluble. These are not stored in the body, but are discharged from the kidneys in urine. They are sensitive to strong light and heat, and are destroyed by boiling. Vitamin C is rapidly lost from a cut surface when exposed to the air, as oxygen absorbs it.

Table I.—Sources and Functions of Vitamins

VITAMIN	SOURCES	FUNCTIONS
A	Fish-liver oils, dairy produce, eggs, carrots, and green vegetables	Growth of sight
B-complex	Yeast, peanuts, bacon, ham, wholemeal bread, green peas, liver, cabbage, milk, Marmite	Oxidation of sugar, nutrition of nerves, health of skin and mucosa, manufacture of red blood-cells. Exact action depends on which member of B-complex is concerned
C (ascorbic acid)	Fresh fruit and vegetables	Aids resistance to infections, plays a part in growth, and in wound and bone healing
D	Fish-liver oils, animal fats, margarine, sardine, egg	Concerned in utilization of calcium and phosphorus for teeth and bones
E	Milk, wheat-germ	Might prevent abortion
K	Cabbage, green peas	Essential for normal clotting

For a well-balanced diet one should eat something of each type of food daily. The energy requirement varies with occupation and other energy outlets. If more food is eaten than needed for energy expended, the rest is often stored as fat and the person puts on weight. Alcohol and carbohydrates add a great deal of weight. Thus the secret of reducing weight is only to eat sufficient food for the actual energy requirement. But slimming diets can be dangerous unless under medical supervision.

EXCRETION

Elimination of water and waste products of metabolism; via kidneys, skin, bowels, and lungs.

Kidneys

These lie in the upper part of the abdomen, one on each side of the lumbar vertebrae. From each arises a long tube (ureter) which carries urine containing waste products to the storage reservoir (bladder), which lies low in the pelvis. When the bladder is full, pressure forces open the sphincter muscle, allowing the urine to pass into another tube (urethra), which carries it outside the body.

The kidneys consist of thousands of tiny (uriniferous) tubules. These are surrounded by a network of capillaries, from which they receive waste products from the blood.

FUNCTIONS OF KIDNEYS

1. Excretion of waste material and water.
2. Elimination of drugs which have passed through the body circulation.
3. Regulation of composition of blood plasma.
4. Partial control of sugar content of blood.

If the kidneys fail to excrete sufficient water, an excess remains in the blood-stream; this passes out into the tissues, causing swelling (oedema). This readily occurs in legs and eyelids. When pressed the skin may remain depressed for a while (pitting oedema).

Toxaemia is retention of waste products of metabolism, which causes a poisoning effect.

On top of each kidney is a suprarenal gland, which secretes adrenalin. The latter:—

a. Stimulates actions of involuntary muscles.
b. Releases glycogen from the liver.
c. Increases blood-sugar.
d. Acts as a haemostat to stop bleeding.

The Skin

The epidermis (outer layer of cells) is constantly being shed due to friction. Below is the dermis. In this layer lie tiny nerve-endings, capillaries, hair follicles, sweat, and sebaceous glands.

FUNCTIONS OF SKIN

1. Protection against entry of (a) organisms and (b) water (skin is waterproof).
2. Excretion of water and unwanted products of metabolism. Up to 1 pint (600 ml.) can be lost in one day.
3. Control of body temperature.

With raised body temperature the pores of the skin open and sweat glands pour out their secretions. These evaporate from the body and cool the surface. At the same time extra skin capillaries open out, allowing more blood to flow near the surface, where it loses its heat.

With cold, skin vessels close down to give the surface a bluish appearance, more of the deeper veins showing through. At the same time contraction of tiny muscles at the base of skin hairs causes them to stand up on end (goose-pimple effect). This traps a tiny amount of warm air close to the skin. Shivering may occur, this consisting of violent muscle movements which generate heat.

MEASUREMENT OF BODY TEMPERATURE

This is measured with a clinical thermometer, which is a glass tube expanded into a bulb at one end. Mercury in this bulb expands with heat, forcing the mercury to move up the tube, against measurements etched on to the glass. We are thus in a position to know the temperature around the bulb. At the top of the bulb a small crook prevents mercury returning to the bulb until the thermometer is shaken.

Normal body temperature is 98·4° Fahrenheit or 37° Centigrade. It tends to be lower in the morning and higher in the afternoon. It changes with shock, lack of food, and illness.

Registration of Temperature

1. In the mouth.
2. Under the arm: this tends to be slightly cooler.
3. In the groin: also cooler.
4. In the rectum: this is very useful for young children. In this case the reading is higher than usual.

QUESTIONS

1. Describe the circulation of blood. What important changes occur in the blood during circulation ?
2. What are the functions of blood ? How does it clot ?
3. Give a brief description of the alimentary canal.
4. Discuss briefly:—
    a. Pulmonary artery and vein.
    b. Reasons for using a clinical thermometer.

CHAPTER III

SPECIAL ANATOMY AND PHYSIOLOGY

BEFORE studying dental health and disease it is essential to have a sound understanding of the underlying biological principles. This chapter re-enforces those aspects of anatomy and physiology which are related to the treatment of patients in dental and oral surgery.

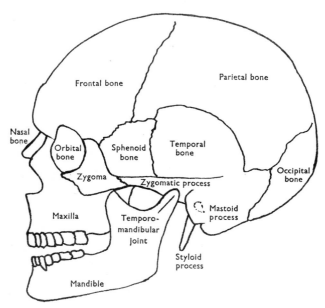

Fig. 9.—Side view of skull.

MORPHOLOGY OF THE SKULL (*Figs.* 9, 10)

This refers to the shape of the bony skeleton of the head and jaws. It consists of two parts, a box-like cranium containing and protecting the brain, and the facial skeleton. Added protection is given to the brain by its surrounding cerebral fluid. The skull rests upon the upper end of the vertebral column. To obtain a clear picture of the position of the bones, students are advised to look at a skull for study purposes. Dentists sometimes have one at the surgery.

THE CRANIUM CONSISTS OF 8 BONES

    1 frontal bone forms the forehead.
    2 parietal bones form the side of skull.
    2 temporal bones contain the ears.
    1 occipital bone forms base of skull.
    1 sphenoid bone ⎫
    1 ethmoid bone ⎭ these form the floor of the cranium.

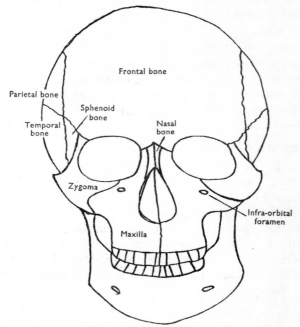

Fig. 10.—Front view of skull.

THE FACE CONSISTS OF 14 BONES

    2 lacrymal bones ⎫
    2 nasal bones   ⎬ These form the nose.
    2 turbinate (conchae) bones
    1 vomer bone ⎭
    1 mandible
    2 maxillary bones.
    2 palatine bones.
    2 zygomatic (malar) bones.

The four maxillary and zygomatic bones form the upper jaw, in close association with the palatine bones.

The mandible (lower jaw) is the only mobile bone in the skull: it articulates with the temporal bone on each side of the cranium by means of a temporomandibular joint, to allow for the movements involved in mastication. All other bones are joined by normal sutures, which aid growth of the skull.

Foramen Magnum

Large opening in the base of the cranium for passage of the spinal cord from the brain.

THE MAXILLARY BONES (*Fig.* 11)

The main bones of the facial skeleton, there being one for each side. They meet in the midline of the face, below the nose, and together form the upper jaw. Each maxilla consists of a body and four processes; alveolar, palatine, frontal, and zygomatic.

The *body* has four surfaces and a large central cavity or antrum:—

1. THE ANTERIOR OR FACIAL SURFACE

Above, it forms part of the lower margin of the orbit, beneath which is the infra-orbital foramen. This is the exit for the infra-orbital nerves and vessels.

Laterally is the zygomatic process.

Below, it is continuous with the alveolar process.

Medially it forms the side of the front opening to the nose.

Some muscles of facial expression are attached to this surface. It is separated from the posterior surface by the zygomatic process.

2. THE POSTERIOR SURFACE

Forms the anterior wall of the infratemporal fossa, where branches of the maxillary nerve and vessels enter the maxilla via dental canals.

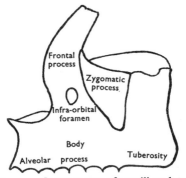

Fig. 11.—Outer aspect of maxillary bone.

To its sides are the zygomatic processes, with the alveolar processes below. The buccinator muscles are attached to this surface above the level of the molar roots.

3. THE SUPERIOR SURFACE

Forms part of the floor of the orbit, below which runs the infra-orbital canal, with its nerves and blood-vessels. It also provides a roof for the antrum.

4. THE MEDIAL SURFACE

Forms the wall of the nose. An opening (maxillary hiatus) allows fluid to pass from the antrum into the nose. In front of this hiatus is the nasolacrimal duct (tear-duct) bringing fluid from the eye.

Bones in Contact with the Maxilla

Maxilla of the opposite side.
Ethmoid.
Frontal.
Inferior concha and vomer.
Lacrimal.
Mandible.
Nasal.
Palatine.

Muscles attached to the Maxillary Bone

Buccinator.
Compressor nares.
Dilator nares.
Inferior oblique of eye and inferior rectus.
Levator anguli oris (caninis).
Levator labii superioris.
Levator labii superioris alequae nasi.
Masseter.
Medial pterygoid.
Orbicularis oculi.
Orbicularis oris.
Zygomaticus.

THE PALATE (*Fig.* 12)

Consists of an anterior hard portion, and a posterior soft part. Above is the nose, and below are the mouth and pharynx.

Hard Palate

Consists of bone covered by mucosa tightly bound to bone (muco-periosteum). It is formed by two palatine processes of the maxillae anteriorly, and two horizontal plates of palatine bone posteriorly. It is bounded in front and at the sides by the horseshoe-shaped alveolar process bearing the teeth. The incisive foramen lies in the midline,

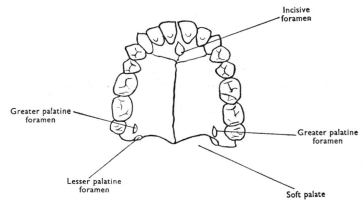

Fig. 12.—The palate, showing foramina or exit for nerves.

just behind the incisors. Through this pass the long sphenopalatine (nasopalatine) nerves and blood-vessels. The greater palatine foramen lies at the junction of palatine and maxillary bones, and transmits the greater palatine nerve and artery. These run forward along a groove between the palate and alveolus. The lesser palatine foramen lies just behind the greater palatine foramen, and transmits the lesser palatine vessels and nerves.

Soft Palate

A muscular mass covered by mucosa above and below. In front it joins the hard palate. Posteriorly it hangs downward as the midline uvula.

During breathing the soft palate is relaxed. However, during deglutition it is firm, lying tightly against the posterior pharyngeal wall, to prevent passage of food to the nose.

THE MAXILLARY ANTRUM OR SINUS

A bony cavity of unknown function within the body of the maxilla. It is one of four air sinuses that communicate with the nose. Its base is formed by the alveolar process, with the tooth roots lying in close approximation. Because of this, any dental infection in the area is liable to spread into the antrum. The antral floor is sometimes broken during tooth extraction, the resulting hole from mouth to antrum being known as an ' oro-antral fistula '.

THE MANDIBLE (*Fig.* 13)

Formed by two bones united in the midline (symphysis menti). Each consists of a horizontal horseshoe-shaped body and a laterally placed vertical ramus.

The Body

On top, the teeth lie in sockets within the alveolar process. Below the roots of the premolar teeth the mental foramen transmits the mental

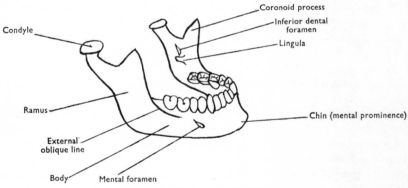

Fig. 13.—The mandible.

nerve and vessels through the outer surface. Passing back and slightly upwards from this foramen is the external oblique line, which becomes continuous with the anterior border of the ramus. Above this line lie the tooth roots. Below is the inferior dental canal. Near the midline on the lower border is a small digastric depression or fossa, from which arises the anterior belly of the digastric muscle. The outer surface of the mandible provides attachment for several muscles of facial expression and of mastication. The buccinator muscle is attached buccally to the lower molar teeth.

On the lingual aspect the mylohyoid line runs down and forwards from the region of the third molar tooth to the midline. Below the mylohyoid line a submandibular fossa houses the submandibular salivary gland. Above, the sublingual salivary gland lies in a fossa of the same name. Just above the posterior part of the line the lingual nerve lies on the bone beneath the oral mucous membrane. Below this region the mylohyoid nerve and vessels lie in the corresponding groove.

Ascending Ramus

Has two upward projections, a posterior condyle and an anterior coronoid process. The condyle articulates with the temporal bone as part of the temporomandibular joint, and provides attachment for the lateral pterygoid muscle. To the coronoid is attached the temporal muscle.

The external surface of the ramus is flat, with several oblique ridges. Fibres of masseter muscle are attached to almost the whole side. Behind and above this muscle lies the parotid salivary gland.

The medial pterygoid muscle is attached to a large proportion of the inner aspect of the ascending ramus. Immediately above this, lying approximately half-way along a line between the angle of the mandible and the third molar, is the mandibular foramen, through which the inferior dental nerve and vessels enter the mandibular canal. The entrance to the foramen is overhung by a bony projection, the lingula, to which is attached the sphenomandibular ligament. Below the lingula the mylohyoid groove passes down and forwards on to the body carrying the mylohyoid vessels and nerve.

The posterior and lower borders of the mandible meet at the angle, to which is attached the stylomandibular ligament. The parotid salivary gland lies in contact with the posterior border.

Muscles attached to the Mandible

Anterior belly of the digastric.
Buccinator.
Depressor labii inferioris.
Depressor anguli oris.
Genioglossus.
Geniohyoid.
Lateral pterygoid.
Masseter.
Medial pterygoid.
Mentalis.
Mylohyoid.
Orbicularis oris.
Platysma.
Superior constrictor of pharynx.
Temporalis.

TEMPOROMANDIBULAR JOINT (*Fig.* 14)

Allows movement between the mandibular condyle and temporal fossa. It thus makes possible opening, closing, and all other movements of the mandible.

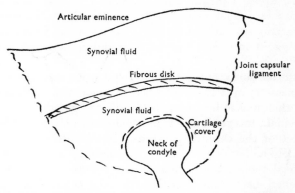

Fig. 14.—Anatomy of temporomandibular joint. The synovial fluid acts as a shock absorber and the fibrous disk allows movements.

The capsular ligament is helped to support the joint in position by two accessory ligaments namely:—

1. Temporomandibular ligament: fibres join back of capsule.
2. Sphenomandibular ligament: attached to side of capsule at point of rotation.

MOVEMENTS OF MANDIBLE (*Fig.* 15)

1. *Opening:* A mixture of hinged and gliding actions. With initial opening of the mouth the mandible rotates around its condyle within the fossa. Upon further opening the articular disk moves forward on the articular eminence, followed by rotation of the condyle on the lower surface of the disk. These opening movements are carried out by means of both lateral pterygoid muscles, the mylohyoid, digastric and infra-hyoid muscles, all acting together. The first named pull condyle and disk forward, whilst the rest depress the mandible.

2. *Closure:* Contraction of the temporalis, masseter, and medial pterygoid muscles on both sides elevates the mandible.

3. *Protrusion:* Contraction of both lateral pterygoid muscles.

4. *Retrusion:* Involves contraction of horizontal fibres of the temporalis muscles.

5. *Sideways movements:* Contraction of some fibres of the medial pterygoids.

6. *Chewing:* Anterior, posterior, and lateral movements. Alternate action of the lateral pterygoids and temporalis muscles on the same side

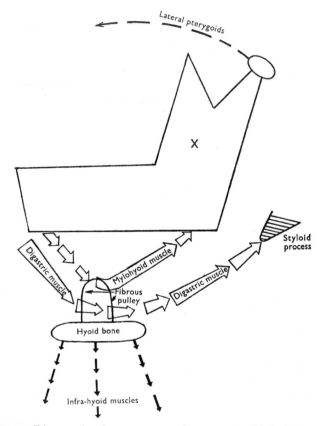

Fig. 15.—Diagram showing movements of temporomandibular joint. Lateral pterygoids pull condyle forward whilst digastric and mylohyoid muscles pull mandible downwards, to rotate around the entrance to the inferior dental canal (X).

leads to protrusion and retrusion of that side, with the chin going to the opposite side.

MUSCLES OF MASTICATION

These muscles are all innervated by the mandibular division of the trigeminal nerve.

DESCRIPTION OF INDIVIDUAL MUSCLES

1. *Digastrics:* Lie anteriorly and posteriorly below the mandible to form part of the floor of the mouth. They are attached to the hyoid bone, mandible, and maxilla. They elevate and retract the tongue and hyoid bone.

2. *Masseter:* Broad muscle attached to the zygomatic arch bone and the angle of the mandible. It is very powerful and exerts great pressure during chewing. It draws the mandible upwards.

3. *Temporalis:* Fan-shaped muscle which spreads out from the temporal bone on either side of the skull. It is also attached to the coronoid process of the mandible and assists in closing the mouth.

4. *Pterygoids:* These are deeply embedded within the cheeks and are attached to the sphenoid bone and the mandible. They raise and draw forward the mandible and take part in chewing movements.

MUSCLE	ACTION
Digastric	Opens mouth
Infrahyoids	Pull mandible down
Masseter	Closes mouth
Temporalis	Closes mouth and retracts mandible
Medial pterygoid	Raises and draws mandible forward
Lateral pterygoid	Draws mandible and disc forward

MUSCLES OF FACIAL EXPRESSION

This group of muscles gives rise to the characteristic expressions seen on the face, such as frowning and laughing. It includes all the muscles of the nose, cheeks, mouth, and forehead, as well as the external muscles of the eyes. The main ones are as follows:—

1. *Buccinator (Trumpeter's Muscle):* The muscle plane of each cheek. It provides power for sucking and blowing, e.g., whilst playing wind instruments. During chewing it keeps food in contact with the teeth.

It is attached to the outer aspects of the alveolar processes of maxilla and mandible opposite the molar teeth. In front many fibres join the orbicularis oris, and behind they join the muscles of the pharynx at the pterygomandibular raphe. The buccinator is pierced opposite the upper molars by Stenson's (parotid) duct.

2. *Orbicularis Oris:* Forms the mass of the lips. Contraction leads to closure of the anterior opening of the mouth. Accessory muscles alter its position.

3. *Orbicularis Oculi:* A sphincter muscle which protects the eyeball and other orbital contents. It keeps the eyeball cleansed with tears, which sweep away dust and other particles.

4. *Frontalis:* The muscle which produces characteristic wrinkling of the forehead.

GROWTH OF THE SKULL

This occurs in one or more of three ways:—

1. *Sutural Growth:* With growth of underlying organs such as the brain or eyeball, sutures between bones are stretched and fresh bone is laid down in the area between the bones. This process slows down after the age of about seven years. An example is growth between the maxilla and its neighbours.

2. *Cartilaginous Growth:* In some regions growth takes place by an increase in size of cartilage, which is then replaced by bone. This type of growth takes place in the mandibular condyle.

3. *Surface Deposition:* In some places further bone is deposited on the surface of existing bone, growth taking place in the direction of deposition. In order to prevent gross increase in thickness of the part, this deposition is often associated with bone resorption elsewhere. Such growth is apparent in both jaws.

THE ORAL CAVITY

This is surrounded by the soft and hard palate above, the cheeks to the sides, lips to the front, and pharynx at the back. Below are the structures of the floor of the mouth, the greater part of which is formed by the tongue.

Vestibule: Space bounded externally by the lips and cheeks and internally by the gums and teeth.

Hard Palate: Composed of processes of the maxilla and palatine bones.

Soft Palate: Movable fold of mucous membrane suspended from the back of the hard palate. It encloses muscles, blood-vessels, nerves, and mucous glands. Hanging from the centre of its posterior border is the conical shaped uvula.

Fauces: An aperture leading from mouth to pharynx. It commences on either side of the uvula as a curved fold of muscular tissue covered by mucous membrane. It divides into two parts: (1) The anterior pillar of fauces which passes down, out, and forward to the side of the base of the tongue; (2) The posterior pillar of fauces which passes down and back to the side of the pharynx.

Tonsils: Two lymphoid glands, one on either side of the pharynx. They act as filters and prevent organisms from food and other sources being swallowed. They contain deep crypts in which infection may lodge.

Pharynx: A muscular tube lined with mucous membrane. It is cone-shaped, with its broad end at the base of the skull. Two openings at the back of the nasal cavity (posterior nares) connect pharynx and nose. Below, it continues as the oesophagus.

Nasopharynx: Lies behind the nose and above the soft palate. On its lateral walls are two openings, the Eustachian (auditory) tubes. These are in direct communication with the middle ears, to which they convey air.

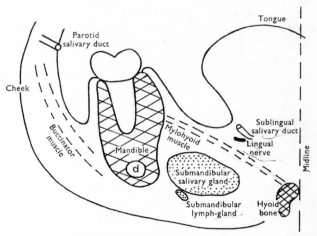

Fig. 16.—Section through the lower jaw showing relations of mandible and tongue. d, inferior dental canal for nerves and blood-vessels.

Oropharynx: That part of pharynx lying behind the mouth and below the soft palate.

Laryngopharynx: Extends from the oropharynx to the oesophagus; thus from the level of the second cervical vertebra to the sixth cervical vertebra.

FLOOR OF THE MOUTH (*Fig.* 16)

Formed basically by the mylohyoid muscle, on which lies the tongue. The mylohyoid originates from the mylohyoid line on the inner aspect of each side of the mandible. This line runs forward from the last molar tooth to the symphysis menti. In the midline, posterior muscle fibres hang down to reach the hyoid bone, the rest forming a free posterior border which is partially covered by the submandibular salivary glands. Several important branches of the mandibular nerves and vessels pass over and below the muscle.

Mylohyoid

Forms a muscular basis for the floor of the mouth. Upon contraction it lifts up the hyoid bone and the root of the tongue. If the hyoid bone is fixed, contraction of the mylohyoid pulls down the mandible to assist in opening the mouth.

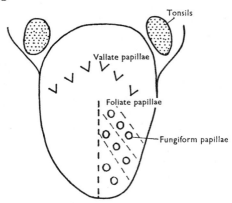

Fig. 17.—The surface of the tongue.

THE TONGUE

A highly muscular structure lying on the floor of the mouth and covered by mucous membrane (*Fig.* 17). The upper surface mucosa is covered with taste-buds, which are knob-like projections lying within the epithelial tissue and containing the organs of taste. The large buds (vallate papillae) are arranged in V-shaped rows at the back of the tongue. The smaller filiform and fungiform papillae are distributed over the surface and sides of the tongue. The posterior part is more smooth and regular and has a few swellings of lymph tissue, the lingual tonsil.

The Muscular Organ of the Tongue (*Fig.* 18)

The main muscles are the two genioglossus muscles. Within their substance a mass of *intrinsic* muscles lead to various changes of shape. They are divided into longitudinal, vertical, and horizontal fibres.

Extrinsic muscles are attached to the tongue, altering its position within the mouth. These include the hyoglossus, palatoglossus, and styloglossus. Intrinsic and extrinsic muscles act together in speech, mastication, and deglutition.

Genioglossus: Arises from the genial tubercles in the midline of the mandible. Contraction leads to protrusion of the tongue, with its tip tending to go towards the opposite side.

Hyoglossus: Extends from the hyoid bone to the tongue. It depresses and retracts the side of the tongue.

Palatoglossus: Runs down from the palate just in front of the tonsil to form the anterior pillar of the fauces. It approximates the back of the tongue and soft palate during swallowing movements.

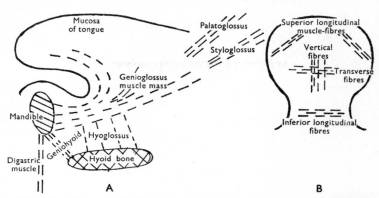

Fig. 18.—Diagrams showing the structure of the tongue. A, Extrinsic view seen from the side, showing structures attached to the outside of the main genioglossus muscle mass. B, Intrinsic diagram showing inside of tongue looking from in front of the mouth.

Styloglossus: Fibres from the styloid process pull the sides of the tongue up and back.

Functions of the Tongue

Mastication.
Swallowing (deglutition).
Speech.
Detection of:—
　Taste.
　Pain.
　Touch.
　Pressure.
　Temperature.

Taste is a chemical sensation, so solid substances must first be dissolved in water or saliva before they can be analysed by the senses. Sour taste is received at the sides of the tongue, bitter at the back, and sweet and salt at its tip.

THE HYOID BONE

This is shaped like a horse-shoe and lies in the neck, above the larynx (voice box) and below the mandible. It is connected to the styloid process of the temporal bone by the stylohoid muscle, and to the tongue by the hyoglossus muscle. It does not articulate with any other bones.

The hyoid consists of (a) a body which forms its central part; (b) the greater and lesser cornu which form two projections on each side of the body.

The bone can be felt in the neck just above the laryngeal prominence (Adam's apple). Its main function is to give support to the tongue, and attachment to some of its muscles.

MASTICATION (CHEWING)

Preparation of food for swallowing. The teeth incise and chew food in to small pieces, which are then moistened and partially digested by saliva. Stimulation of taste-buds and the sight of attractively served food cause increased salivary flow. The tongue and cheeks keep food in contact with the teeth.

DEGLUTITION (SWALLOWING)

Passage of food from mouth to pharynx.

In order to prevent food passing into the nose, the nasopharynx is sealed off by approximation of soft palate to back of pharynx. The larynx is sealed off by the epiglottis.

Swallowing is carried out by contraction of mylohyoid, digastric, stylohyoid, styloglossus, and palatoglossus muscles, which raise the tongue towards the palate. Contraction of its intrinsic muscles leads to alterations in shape of the tongue, forcing the bolus (softened mass of food) towards the pharynx. At this point the pharyngeal constrictor muscles propel the food downwards into the oesophagus, from where it passes to the stomach.

SALIVARY GLANDS

The main salivary glands are paired, one on each side.
1. Parotid glands, with Stenson's ducts (in the cheeks).
2. Submandibular, with Wharton's ducts (beneath the mandible).
3. Sublingual, with many small ducts (below the tongue).

1. Parotid

A pyramidal-shaped gland lying below the ear and behind the angle of the mandible. Some of it projects forward over the masseter. As the gland is contained within a restricting fascial sheath, there is much tension and pain with inflammation and swelling (e.g., in mumps). Saliva escapes to the mouth via Stenson's ducts which lie opposite the maxillary second molars.

2. Submandibular

This gland lies against the inner aspects of the mandible, close to the molars and premolars. As it curves around the posterior border of the mylohyoid muscle some of the gland lies within the mouth and some in the neck. Wharton's ducts open via papillae to the floor of the mouth, below the tongue.

3. Sublingual

Lies beneath the mucosa of the floor of the mouth at the side of the lingual fraenum, in contact with the sublingual fossa (depression) on the inner surface of the mandible, close to the symphysis menti. Just behind is the deep part of the submandibular gland. It has fifteen to twenty ducts, some of which open direct to the oral cavity by sublingual papillae and some via the submandibular papillae.

SALIVA

Fluid secreted by salivary glands.

Constituents

90 per cent water.
Calcium carbonate and calcium phosphates (maintain alkalinity).
Carbon dioxide.
Oxygen.
Enzymes, e.g., amylase (ptyalin), maltase.
Mucin (from submandibular and sublingual glands).

Functions

1. *Digestion:* Amylase begins breakdown of food starches to the simple sugar maltose. Maltase converts maltose to glucose.

2. *Bolus formation:* Softening of food by incorporation of moisture makes it easier to swallow.

3. *Lubrication:* Assists passage of bolus and keeps mouth and lips soft, this aiding clear speech.

4. *Cleansing action:* The constant flow washes and cleans the mouth and teeth removing food debris, old epithelial cells and foreign particles. Also saliva inhibits the growth of bacterial organisms by removing substances which aid their nutrition and growth.

5. *Excretory:* Many substances are removed via saliva, e.g., ketones from diabetics.

6. *Alkalinity:* Amylase only acts in a neutral or alkaline environment.

7. *Solvent action:* As taste is a chemical sense, solids must be dissolved before they can be tasted.

Volume

1. In health, normally about two pints per day.
2. Feverish illnesses cause depression of salivary secretion with subsequent dry mouth, stagnation, and decomposition of organic material. Swarms of bacteria collect on the teeth and lips unless this organic film is removed by artificial means, e.g., by wiping with toothbrush or moistened gauze.
3. Nervousness leads to inhibition of salivary secretion with drying of the mouth and lips (public speakers often sip water).
4. Teething produces extra saliva, much of which dribbles on to the infant's chin. If left the warm moisture encourages growth of organisms.

NOSE AND NASAL CAVITY

The nasal cavity is the first organ of respiration. Its roof is formed from the base of the skull, and its floor by the roof of the mouth. The large irregular-shaped cavity is divided by a midline septum into two nostrils. This medial septum consists of a perpendicular plate of the ethmoid above, and the vomer below. Cartilage forms the mass of the nose and is continuous with the nasal bones.

Inside the nostrils the lateral walls are scroll-shaped, providing increased areas of membrane tissue with copious capillary blood-vessels to supply warmth to the incoming air. This membrane tissue is also well supplied with hair-like cilia to prevent dust and organisms entering the air-passages. The membrane lining is kept moist by special cells.

OPENINGS INTO THE NASAL CAVITY

1. Anterior nares through which air passes from the exterior.
2. Posterior nares to the nasopharynx.
3. Lateral openings (ostia) to the maxillary sinuses.
4. Upper lateral openings to the ethmoidal sinuses.
5. Openings to the frontal and sphenoidal sinuses.

Functions of the Nose

1. Smell.
2. Intake of oxygenated air.
3. Expiration of de-oxygenated air.
4. Filtration of air by cilia trapping foreign bodies.
5. Sneezing to remove trapped foreign bodies, which are thus not inhaled.

SMELL

The first pair of cranial nerves (olfactory) convey the sense of smell. Nerve-fibres from the upper section of the nose pass upwards through the ethmoid bones, to the group of nerve-cells known as the ' olfactory bulb '. Stimuli are thus conveyed to an area of smell reception at the base of the brain.

THE SINUSES

These are spaces within the skull bones which reduce their weight. Their true function is unknown. They have some influence on voice production, giving it resonance. All except the large maxillary sinuses are near to the central line of the skull when this is viewed from the front.

The mucous membrane lining the sinuses is an extension of the nasal membrane. Thus any infection or inflammation easily spreads

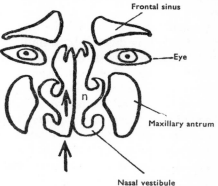

Fig. 19.—Front view of nasal cavities (n) showing their relationship to eyes, frontal sinuses, maxillary antrum, and nasal vestibule. Arrows show the direction taken by inhaled air.

between them, causing sinusitis. Behind the ear in the temporal bone are mastoid cells, comparable in structure to the sinuses. These are also lined with an extension of their mucous membrane, which makes the mastoid areas very vulnerable to infection.

Four pairs of air sinuses communicate with the nasal cavity (*Fig.* 19):—

1. Frontal ⎫
2. Ethmoid ⎬ Open into the nasal cavity.

3. Sphenoid: Opens to the naso-pharynx.

4. Maxillary antra of Highmore: Each antrum opens to the lateral wall of the nasal passage. They are very large, and lie above the roots of maxillary canines, premolars and molars.

CRANIAL NERVES

Twelve pairs emerge directly from the brain; some nerves are purely sensory, others are motor, and some are mixed.

Sensory: Receive external stimuli and pass the message to the brain, e.g., carry sensations of pain, temperature, and pressure.

Motor: Carry messages from brain to area of action. Muscles or organs then react by movement or secretion.

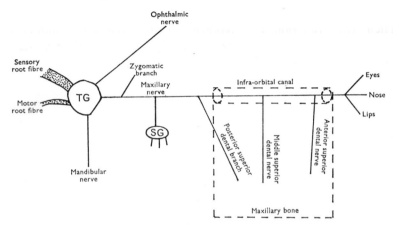

Fig. 20.—Diagram showing how trigeminal ganglion (TG) gives off three nerves; the ophthalmic, maxillary, and mandibular nerves. The ganglion receives sensory and motor root fibres. The maxillary nerve gives off zygomatic and posterior superior dental branches before entering the infra-orbital canal of the maxillary bone, where it is known as the 'infra-orbital nerve'. The middle and anterior superior dental nerves are given off from the infra-orbital nerve whilst it is still within the canal. It then passes out of the foramen and sends fibres to skin around the eyes, nose, and lips. Fibres from the main maxillary nerve pass to the sphenopalatine ganglion (SG).

Mixed: Carry messages to and from the brain, the one nerve therefore doing all the necessary work required for muscle or organ response.

Nerves of the Head and Face

Sensory and motor innervation of this part of the body is mainly by branches of the fifth (trigeminal) and seventh (facial) cranial nerves, which are both mixed nerves.

TRIGEMINAL NERVE

This is divided into three divisions, the first two being sensory only whilst the third carries motor and sensory fibres.

Sensory fibres pass from the skin of the face and forehead, eyes, nose, part of the outer ear, tympanic membrane (ear-drum), oral mucous membrane, tongue, gingivae, periodontal membrane, and teeth.

Motor fibres supply the muscles of mastication, tensor palati, and tensor tympani of the ear.

1. *Ophthalmic Division (sensory only):—*

a. Lacrimal gland.

b. Upper eyelid, upper nasal skin, and mucosa.

c. Top of scalp, forehead, conjunctiva, anterior two-thirds side of nose to tip.

2. *Maxillary Division (sensory only) (Fig. 20):—*

a. Upper teeth and their periodontal membranes.

b. Mucous membrane of the upper jaw and cheek, gingivae, soft and hard palate, tonsil, part of nose.

c. Skin of lower eyelid, posterior part of side of nose, upper lip, anterior and upper cheek, lower and anterior part of temporal region, and side of orbit.

Sphenopalatine ganglion (Fig. 21): A circular enlargement of nervous tissue suspended from the maxillary nerve close to its origin. It gives rise to the greater and lesser palatine, and the naso-palatine nerves.

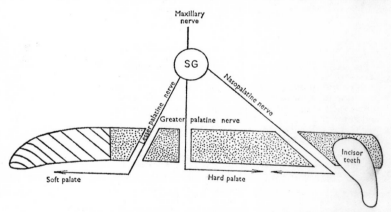

Fig. 21.—Section through the palate showing how the sphenopalatine ganglion (SG), which itself comes from the maxillary nerve, gives off nerves to the soft and hard palates. The long sphenopalatine or nasopalatine nerve comes out through a foramen in the palate just behind the incisor teeth. The greater palatine leaves via the back of the hard palate. The lesser palatine nerve comes out just behind the greater palatine, but passes back to supply the soft palate.

3. *Mandibular Division (motor and sensory) (Fig. 22):—*

This is the largest branch.

a. Secreto-motor to parotid salivary gland.

b. Secreto-motor to submandibular and sublingual glands, impulses coming from the facial nerve.

c. Mandibular teeth and periodontal membranes.

d. Mucosa of anterior two-thirds of tongue, floor of mouth, lower gum and lip, lower part of cheek.

e. Skin of mandible (except near the parotid) extending up to the external ear and side of head. Also lining of the external auditory meatus.

f. Muscles of mastication, tensor palati and tensor tympani of the ear.

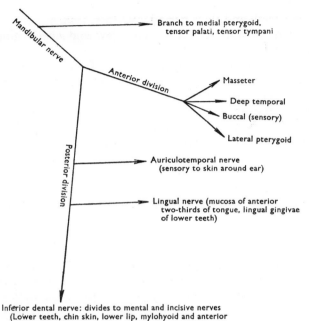

Fig. 22.—The branches of the mandibular division of the trigeminal nerve. Before dividing into anterior and posterior divisions it gives off a small branch to the medial pterygoid, tensor palati, and tensor tympani muscles.

Some Sensory Nerves associated with Local Anaesthesia in Dentistry

1. Inferior dental.
2. Mental.
3. Lingual.
4. Long buccal.
5. Infra-orbital, including middle and anterior superior dental.
6. Posterior superior dental.
7. Greater palatine.

8. Lesser palatine.
9. Nasopalatine.

INFERIOR DENTAL NERVE

A branch of the posterior division of the mandibular nerve. It enters the mandible via a foramen next to the lingula and travels along the mandibular canal close to the roots of the lower teeth. In the premolar region it divides into mental and incisive nerves.

The inferior dental nerve innervates the lower teeth, gingivae, and periodontal membranes, and skin and mucosa of the lower lip and chin. The canine and incisor regions are supplied by the incisive nerve, and the premolar region by the mental nerve. The inferior dental nerve supplies the buccal mucosa and gingivae in the posterior and anterior regions, but the area related to the first molar and second premolar receives fibres from the long buccal nerve.

MENTAL NERVE

This branch of the inferior dental nerve emerges from the mandibular canal via the mental foramen, between the root apices of the lower premolars. It supplies the skin and mucosa of chin and lower lip, and periodontal membranes of the premolars. If anaesthetic solution is passed into the foramen itself the premolars, canines, and incisors will also be anaesthetized.

LINGUAL NERVE

Another branch of the posterior division of the mandibular nerve. It supplies the lingual gingivae and lingual mucosa of the lower jaw, as well as mucosa overlying the anterior two-thirds of the tongue. Therefore when this nerve is anaesthetized prior to the extraction of lower teeth the tongue is also affected.

The lingual nerve also receives fibres from the chorda-tympani branch of the facial nerve, through which it transmits sensations of taste.

LONG BUCCAL NERVE

The only sensory branch of the anterior division of the mandibular nerve. It travels buccally over the mandible, just behind the last molar. It supplies a small area of buccal gingivae and mucosa in the region of the second premolar and first molar, as well as mucosa of cheek.

INFRA-ORBITAL NERVE

After giving off posterior superior dental branches the maxillary nerve enters the infra-orbital canal below the orbit, where it becomes the infra-orbital nerve. It leaves this canal via the infra-orbital foramen below the eye, sending fibres to the skin of the side of the nose, lower eyelids, and upper lip. Within the canal it gives off middle and anterior superior dental nerves, which together with the posterior superior dental nerves form a plexus innervating the upper teeth and periodontal membranes, buccal gingivae, and part of the antral lining.

POSTERIOR SUPERIOR DENTAL NERVE

A small nerve that leaves the maxillary nerve before the latter enters the infra-orbital canal. It runs down the posterior aspect of the maxilla and then enters the bone, where it joins the above mentioned plexus.

GREATER PALATINE NERVE

A branch from the sphenopalatine ganglion. It leaves the bone via a foramen in the bony palate and passes forward to supply the palatal mucosa and gingivae as far forward as the upper canine.

LESSER PALATINE NERVE

This also comes from the above ganglion. It leaves via a foramen just behind the greater palatine foramen, and passes backwards to supply sensory fibres to the soft palate.

NASOPALATINE (LONG SPHENOPALATINE) NERVE

After leaving the sphenopalatine ganglion this nerve passes down alongside the medial aspect of the nose leaving the bone via a foramen behind the maxillary incisors. The nerve supplies palatal mucosa and gingivae as far back as the canines.

The Facial Nerve

This consists of two parts. The main nerve goes to the muscles of facial expression, the posterior belly of the digastric muscle, and the stylohyoid muscle.

The minor portion contains sensory fibres from the face as well as taste-fibres from the anterior two-thirds of the tongue and palate. Sensory branches are given off to the temporal, zygomatic, buccal, mandibular, and cervical regions. Taste fibres are carried in a branch known as the chorda tympani, which reaches taste-buds on the tongue via the lingual nerve.

BLOOD VASCULAR SYSTEM

In general the blood-vessels of the head and neck follow the pathways taken by nerves. The two principal arteries are the common carotids. These pass upwards, one on each side of the neck. They divide by the angle of the mandible into external and internal carotid arteries.

    1. *Internal Carotids:* Supply the brain.

    2. *External Carotids:* Supply the head, neck, face, tongue, and teeth. They give off branches as follows:—

    a. Superior thyroid.

    b. Ascending pharyngeal.

    c. Lingual.

    d. Facial.

    e. Occipital.

    f. Posterior auricular.

    g. Superficial temporal (includes parotid gland, temporomandibular joint).

    h. Maxillary (to upper and lower jaws, teeth and periodontal membranes, muscles of mastication, palate, nose).

LYMPH SYSTEM OF THE HEAD AND NECK

Fluid from this part of the body eventually drains to cervical lymph-glands on each side of the neck, but first travels through one or more of a ring of nodes encircling the head. Drainage is through glands and ducts on the same side of the midline of the body.

Waldeyer's Ring

A circle of lymph-tissue protecting the entrances to the alimentary and respiratory tracts. It consists of:—

    1. *The Tonsils:* One on each side of the throat.

    2. *The Adenoids:* In the roof of the pharynx.

    3. *Lingual Tonsil:* A small swelling on the back of the tongue.

    4. *Tubal Tonsil:* At the entrances to the Eustachian tubes.

Some Important Groups of Lymph-glands of the Head and Neck

Head	Neck
Occipital	Submandibular
Auricular	Submental
Parotid	Superficial cervical
Facial	Deep cervical

1. SUPERFICIAL CERVICAL

Situated in the upper region of the neck below the angle of the mandible. They drain the ear lobes and skin in this region, as well as the auricular nodes.

2. DEEP CERVICAL

Lie along the carotid sheath as a continuous chain from the base of the skull to the root of the neck. They are divided into upper and lower sections by the omohyoid muscle. These glands drain the base of tongue and sublingual region, posterior palate, and auricular, submental, submandibular and occipital nodes.

3. SUBMANDIBULAR

Situated beneath the inner aspect of the angle of mandible. They drain:—
   a. Upper and lower teeth, except for the lower incisors.
   b. Upper and lower lips, except for the middle part of the lower lip.
   c. Anterior parts of nasal cavity and palate.
   d. Body of the tongue.
Their own outflow passes to the deep cervical glands.

4. SUBMENTAL

In the midline below the chin. They drain:—
   a. Middle of lower lip.
   b. Skin of chin.
   c. Tip of tongue.
   d. Lower incisors and gingivae.
They empty to the submandibular and upper deep cervical glands.

5. FACIAL

Along the facial vein close to the corner of the mouth. They drain the skin over the root of the nose, central forehead, and face. Outflow is to the mandibular gland.

6. PAROTID

Lie in close relationship to the salivary glands. They drain the side of scalp and face, and the eyelids. Outflow is to the upper deep cervical glands.

7. AURICULAR

Consists of several nodes around the ear. They drain the ear and some of the scalp. Outflow is to the superficial cervical and upper deep cervical glands.

8. OCCIPITAL

Lie at the back of the head, which they drain. They swell during German measles (rubella).

Drainage of Specific Regions

1. Lateral surface of head and most of forehead: auricular glands.
2. Middle part of forehead: vessels follow facial vessels to submandibular glands.
3. Eyelids, external nose, upper lip and cheek: submandibular glands.
4. Lower lip and chin: submental and submandibular glands.

Thus the whole of the head, skin and superficial soft tissues drain to the upper deep cervical glands.

5. Nose:—(a) Posterior region: back to retropharyngeal nodes and then to deep cervical glands; (b) Anterior region: to outer face and submandibular glands.
6. Soft palate and most of hard palate: upper deep cervical glands.
7. Anterior part of hard palate: submandibular glands.
8. Base of tongue: submandibular glands.
9. Body of tongue: submandibular glands.
10. Tip of tongue: submental gland.
11. Teeth and periodontal membrane: submandibular glands except for lower incisors which drain to the submental region.

QUESTIONS

1. Write *brief* notes on the following and indicate where each is situated:—
  a. Parotid gland.
  b. Maxillary antrum.
  c. Inferior dental foramen.
  d. Masseter muscle.
  e. Mylohyoid ridge.
2. Write brief notes on:—
  a. The muscles of mastication.
  b. The nerve-supply to the teeth.
3. Describe and illustrate the mandible, its movements in relation to the maxilla, and the muscles which are involved.
4. Describe the following structures and explain their significance in relation to dental treatment:—
  a. Hard Palate.
  b. Soft Palate.

CHAPTER IV

THE ORAL TISSUES

DEVELOPMENT AND GROWTH OF THE FACE AND JAWS

THE whole body develops from three basic embryonic layers: endoderm, mesoderm, and ectoderm. These give rise to the various tissues and organs.

The structures of the face develop when several processes form around the embryonic mouth, come together, and join. Occasionally something goes wrong to prevent them from meeting, resulting in congenital deformities such as hare lip and cleft palate. After the processes have united, the basic embryonic layers differentiate to form the various tissues.

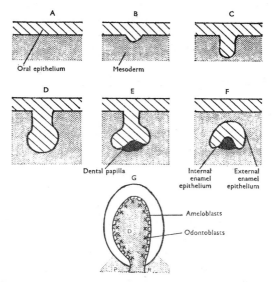

Fig. 23.—Stages in the development of a tooth. A, Mesoderm is covered by oral epithelium. B, C, Epithelium grows down into mesoderm. D, Ballooning of downgrowth. E, Thickening of mesoderm as dental papilla, stopping downgrowth at that point and causing formation of cap shape. F, Enamel organ epithelium loses contact with oral epithelium. G, Inner layer of enamel epithelium forms ameloblasts, which lay down enamel. Outer layer of dental papilla forms odontoblasts, which lay down dentine. A downward growth (R) develops into the root. A thickening (P) of mesoderm develops into the periodontal membrane.

DEVELOPMENT OF THE TEETH AND ASSOCIATED STRUCTURES

Morphodifferentiation (Development of Tooth Shape)

Both ectoderm and mesoderm are concerned in the development of dental structures. The former gives rise to epithelial cells, some of which line the oral cavity and lie on a layer of mesoderm. Oral epithelium and mesoderm together develop into the tooth germ, which consists of an enamel organ and a dental papilla (*Fig.* 23).

In about the sixth week of intra-uterine life part of the oral epithelium grows down into the underlying mesoderm and swells as an enamel bud. Mesoderm at the base of the bud thickens, and the bud grows around it. The epithelium in contact with this thickening (dental papilla) is called 'internal enamel epithelium', and the rest is termed 'external enamel epithelium'. Together they form the enamel organ.

In the crown region internal enamel epithelial cells give rise to ameloblasts, which form enamel. Cells of the dental papilla in contact with ameloblasts give rise to odontoblasts, which form dentine. The rest of the papilla gives rise to pulp cells. Outer and inner enamel layers grow down as Hertwig's sheath to outline the root shape, dentine being formed as in the coronal area. Special cells on the inside of the dental follicle form cementoblasts, which deposit cementum around the root dentine. The middle portion of the dental follicle gives rise to the periodontal membrane, and the outer layer becomes incorporated into the surrounding bone, the tooth therefore being supported within its socket.

Calcification (Hardening)

The next stage is hardening, by calcification, when mineral salts are laid down in the soft matrix.

Calcification may be affected by systemic disturbances such as illness and nutritional deficiencies, and by the presence of localized sites of infection. Disturbances of calcification are known as 'hypocalcification', and those of morphodifferentiation as 'hypoplasia'.

CHRONOLOGY OF CALCIFICATION AND ERUPTION (*Table II*)

Deciduous

Calcification begins at approximately 6 months of foetal life. The roots are complete by 1–1½ years after eruption. Teeth are exfoliated or lost from the mouth about 6 months before their permanent successors are due to erupt.

Permanent

Calcification begins approximately 6 years prior to eruption, except for canines which begin 4 months after birth. The roots are completed 3 years after eruption.

There is a great deal of variation, the teeth of girls tending to erupt before those of boys, and mandibular ones before those of the maxilla.

Table II.—CHRONOLOGY OF CALCIFICATION AND ERUPTION OF TEETH

TOOTH	CROWN COMPLETE	ERUPTION
a. *Deciduous*		
Central incisor	2 months	6 months
Lateral incisor	3 months	9 months
Canine	9 months	18 months
First molar	6 months	12 months
Second molar	12 months	24 months
b. *Permanent*		
Central incisor	4 years	7 years
Lateral incisor	5 years	8 years
Canine	6 years	11 years
First premolar	5 years	9 years
Second premolar	6 years	10 years
First molar	5 years	6 years
Second molar	7 years	12 years
Third molar	12 years	18–24 years

Situation at Birth

All the deciduous teeth plus the first permanent molars are partially calcified at birth. At this time the crowns of the deciduous central incisors are one-third calcified, and the laterals one-fifth. The tips of the canines are calcified, as are the occlusal surfaces of the first deciduous molars and the cusps of the second. The mesiobuccal cusps of the first permanent molars are also calcified.

THE HUMAN DENTITION

There are thirty-two teeth in the permanent dentition, and twenty in the deciduous one.

Permanent Dentition

In each quadrant, from the midline back, there are two incisors, one canine, two premolars, and three molars (*Fig.* 24).

INCISORS

Incise or cut food. Their crowns are flattened buccopalatally to form a sharp elongated incisal edge. They are convex buccally and concave lingually, except for the convex cingulum which may be very pronounced in the maxilla. There is a single root. The tooth next to the midline is the central incisor, to the side of which is the lateral.

CANINES (CUSPIDS)

Pierce and hold food. For this purpose the incisal edge consists of mesial and distal edges rising to a single sharp pointed cusp. There is a convex labial surface, a large lingual cingulum, and a long single root.

PREMOLARS (BICUSPIDS)

Assist molars to chew and grind food. They have two cusps, placed buccally and lingually around a central fissure. The cusps are joined mesially and distally by marginal ridges. In the mandible the buccal cusp is larger than the lingual. The maxillary first premolar tends to have two roots, the rest one.

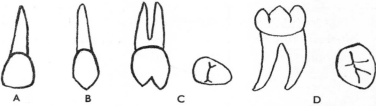

A   B   C   D

Fig. 24.—The permanent teeth. A, Incisor with flat cutting edges. B, Canine with sharp tearing point. C, Upper premolar showing two roots, two cusps, and central fissure. D, Lower molar with two roots, and crown divided by fissures into five cusps.

MOLARS

Chew and grind food. Each has four or five large cusps separated by fissures. The third molars ('wisdom' teeth) are the last to erupt. If there is insufficient room they may become impacted and cause trouble. Upper molars have four cusps; the large mesiopalatal cusp is joined to the distobuccal one by an occlusal ridge, which separates the occlusal depression into two fossae. The distal fossa leads to a palatal fissure. In the lower jaw there are two lingual and two or three buccal cusps around a central branching fissure. The first molar usually has a buccal pit and fissure. The lowers have two, and the uppers three roots.

Deciduous Dentition

This has no premolars, the two deciduous molars occupying the spaces into which the permanent premolars later erupt.

Deciduous teeth tend to be smaller than their permanent successors, with crowns that are more bulbous and whiter. The roots begin from just below the cervical constriction and are very divergent and delicate. The enamel is thin and soft, and the pulps are large and close to the surface.

The second deciduous molars resemble the first permanent molars but are slightly smaller. However, the first ones have a different morphology.

Normal Occlusion (*Fig.* 25)

Ideally the jaws should come together with the teeth in the following relationships:—

1. Buccal cusps and incisive edges of upper teeth occlude buccally to lowers.

2. Upper canines occlude behind lowers.

3. The mesiobuccal cusps of the first maxillary molars occlude with the buccal fissure of the mandibular first molars.

4. Each upper tooth except the last occludes with two lower teeth.

5. There is an overbite of approximately 2 mm.

6. There is an overjet of approximately 2 mm.

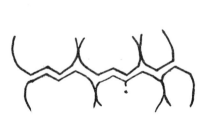 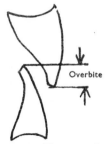

Fig. 25.—Side view of normal relationships between upper and lower teeth. The maxillary molars bite just behind the corresponding lower teeth. The upper incisors come down over the lower ones by an overbite of approximately 2 mm. They also project in front of them by an overjet of about 2 mm.

TEETH

Each tooth consists of a soft central pulp contained in a hard hollow dentine box. The hardness is due to a high proportion of mineral salts. The crown is covered by enamel, and the root by cementum (*Fig.* 26).

The Crown

That part of a tooth which lies in the oral cavity after full eruption has taken place. It is separated from the root by a cervical constriction. The dentine is covered by enamel.

The Root

The portion of a tooth lying within the bony socket, to which it is attached by means of periodontal fibres. The latter are inserted into both alveolar bone and root cementum.

Enamel

The hardest structure in the body. It protects the underlying dentine from external irritants such as masticatory forces, heat and cold,

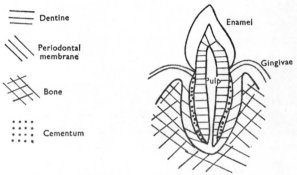

Fig. 26.—A tooth and its surrounding structures.

sweet and sour foods. Enamel is made up of minute highly mineralized prisms.

Cementum

This covers the root dentine. Its main function is attachment of periodontal fibres, and thus support of the tooth within its socket.

Dentine

This forms the mass of a tooth and consists of hollow tubules containing fluid and odontoblast processes. It is these which pass pain impulses to the pulp. Owing to its greater elastic tissue content, dentine is more yielding than enamel, dissipating some of the mechanical shocks applied to a tooth during the course of a lifetime.

Pulp

Soft tissue occupying the pulp chamber in both root (radicular) and crown (coronal). It consists of nerves, blood-vessels, and cells. The main pulp cells are odontoblasts. These lie around the periphery in contact with dentine, which they continue to form throughout life. Odontoblast processes lie in the dentine layer.

ALVEOLAR BONE

A special part of the bone formed when teeth erupt into the mouth, providing a socket for their retention and support. After tooth extraction the alveolus is no longer required; the bone is resorbed and the socket disappears.

PERIODONTAL MEMBRANE (LIGAMENT)

Consists of a mass of fibres which together retain a tooth within its bony socket. They are inserted into both alveolar and bone cementum.

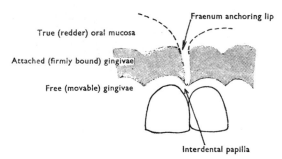

Fig. 27.—The normal oral mucosa.

ORAL MUCOUS MEMBRANE

The covering layer of the mouth. It consists of surface epithelium lying on a deeper connective tissue.

Although generally fairly soft and smooth, the oral epithelium is sometimes modified for special functions. Gums and hard palate have special cornified outer layers to protect them from trauma during mastication. Surface cells are continually shed into the mouth and washed away by saliva. During some illnesses salivary flow decreases and these dead cells collect as a coating (fur) on the tongue. Modifications of tongue mucosa allow the appreciation of taste.

Gingival Mucosa (*Fig.* 27)

Gingival mucosa surrounds the cervical margin of a tooth. It is firmly attached to the underlying bone, except at its free gingival margins. It fills the interproximal regions below contact areas as interdental papillae. In health the attached mucosa is stippled and the free margins are smooth. Loss of this stippling is an early indication of gingivitis. There is no underlying layer of submucosa beneath the stippled portion, the mucosa in this part being firmly bound to underlying bone as mucoperiosteum. There is a similar attachment in most of the hard palate.

Alveolar Mucous Membrane

Normally separated from the attached gingivae by a mucogingival line. Due to the presence of a submucous layer, alveolar mucosa slides freely over the underlying bone.

Fraena

Folds of mucosa labial to the upper and lower incisors, lingual to the lower incisors, and sometimes buccal to the premolars in both jaws. Unless their presence is noted and due allowance made, they impinge on dentures and displace them from position.

QUESTIONS

1. Write notes on the following:—
a. The periodontal membrane.
b. Enamel.
c. Dentine.
d. Functions of the tongue.
e. Deciduous teeth.
f. Lingual fraena.
2. Describe and illustrate the structure of an upper first permanent molar and its relationship to the surrounding structures.
3. Discuss the eruption times of deciduous and permanent teeth.
4. Discuss the functions of teeth.

CHAPTER V

GENERAL PATHOLOGY

Health: A state of maximum physical, mental and social well-being (World Health Organization definition).
Disease: Lack of maximum health.

AETIOLOGY (CAUSATIVE FACTORS OF DISEASE)

Two main groups according to whether they occur before or after birth:—

1. CONGENITAL (BEFORE BIRTH)

   a. Genetic: Certain hereditary conditions such as haemophilia are passed on from generation to generation.

   b. Intra-uterine Infection: When diseases such as German measles are contracted by a woman during the first ten weeks of pregnancy, the developing embryo may be affected, resulting in developmental anomalies such as cleft palate or deafness.

   c. Other Intra-uterine Disturbances: Many drugs taken during pregnancy can affect the developing embryo to cause a malformation of one or more of its parts. An example is thalidomide, which produced many tragic deformities.

2. ACQUIRED (AFTER BIRTH)

   a. Lack of Nourishment: Examples of deficiency diseases are scurvy (lack of vitamin C) and rickets (lack of calcium in the bones). Malnutrition is seldom seen in the United Kingdom.

   b. Infection by Living Organisms: Tuberculosis and syphilis are examples of this type of disease. The degree of infection depends upon the number and virulence of organisms, and the resistance of the host.

   c. Trauma: Examples are gunshot and knife wounds.

   d. Other Physical Damage: Includes radiation and other burns, scalds, and frost-bite.

   e. Chemical Agents: Poisoning and dermatitis.

INFLAMMATION

Those local changes which occur in living tissues when it is injured, providing that the injury is not of such a degree as to destroy at once its structure and vitality.

' Inflammation may be acute or chronic, depending upon the type of irritant and the resistance of the host.

The Acute Inflammatory Reaction

1. At first small blood-vessels dilate or widen to increase the amount of blood flowing through the area.

2. After a few hours blood-flow slows and may even stop. This is due to fluid loss from capillaries to the surrounding tissues, where it remains as an exudate.

3. The blood becomes more viscous (thicker) for the same reason.

4. White blood-cells (leucocytes) are carried along in the centre of blood-vessels, with the red cells (erythrocytes) further out. With slowing of blood-flow they change position. The white cells pass towards, and then through, the vessel walls.

5. During the first 12–24 hours polymorphonuclear leucocytes (neutrophils, acidophils, basophils) leave capillaries for the tissue spaces, to aid defence against irritating substances.

6. Later the mononuclear macrophages (monocytes, lymphocytes, histiocytes) migrate to this site.

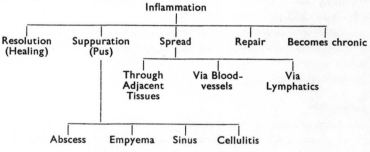

Fig. 28.—Results of acute inflammation.

MECHANISM OF PROTECTION

1. The exudate dilutes toxins to decrease their harmfulness.

2. Antibodies in the exudate assist defence against certain foreign bodies.

3. Phagocytic polymorphs attack and destroy the irritant, forming pus.

4. A fibrin network is laid down, preventing spread of bacteria and other organisms.

CORRELATION OF CLINICAL SIGNS AND SYMPTOMS WITH ACUTE INFLAMMATORY RESPONSES

1. *Redness:* Due to increased blood-flow through the area. Following stasis (stopping of blood-flow), the skin appears bluish.
2. *Heat:* Increased flow brings more internal heat to the surface.
3. *Swelling:* The overlying skin is raised as tissue spaces fill with exudate.
4. *Pain:* Due to pressure and irritation of nerve-endings.
5. *Impaired Function:* Pain and swelling prevent the patient from utilizing that part of the body, allowing it to have a period of rest, and avoiding aggravation of the condition. For example, patients with a painful tooth will carefully chew on the opposite side of the mouth.

SEQUELAE (RESULTS) OF ACUTE INFLAMMATION (*see Fig.* 28)

1. *Resolution:* In those cases involving only mild damage the tissues may return to normal. Pus empties to the lymphatic system, and dead cells are removed by macrophages.
2. *Suppuration:* Formation of pus, the product of fluid exudate and dead cells. It may remain localized or can spread through the tissues:—
a. Abscess: Collection of pus within a confined space.
b. Empyema: Collection of pus in a pre-existing cavity, for example the maxillary antrum.
c. Sinus: Passage of pus from abscess to body surface.
d. Cellulitis: In this case the pus spreads as a diffuse layer through the tissue spaces.
3. *Spread of Infection:*—
a. Through adjacent tissues.
b. Via blood-vessels:—
  i. *Bacteriaemia:* Living organism in blood with no symptoms.
  ii. *Septicaemia:* Spread and multiplication of organisms in the blood-stream causing clinical symptoms.
  iii. *Toxaemia:* Presence in blood of toxins or poisons liberated by bacteria.
c. Via lymphatics: This often causes inflammation and swelling of lymph-glands draining the part. For example, an abscessed lower molar may lead to swelling of the submandibular lymph-gland on that side.
4. *Repair:*—
a. By primary intention: In small non-infected wounds, blood-clot will hold the edges together. Macrophages break down red blood-cells

and fibroblasts then lay down fibres. At the same time new blood-capillaries form. Later, surface epithelium grows over the wound.

b. After infection: In such cases healing occurs from below instead of throughout the tissue. The surface layers remain open (ulcerated) until epithelium grows in from the sides to form a complete covering.

An ulcer—Break in continuity of surface epithelium.

5. *Become Chronic:* This is a slow, smouldering reaction excited in the tissues by mild but injurious agents. It may follow an acute attack or may start as the chronic form, when the irritant is generally a mild physical, chemical, or biological agent. Such a reaction may occur in patients with slightly higher resistance, when there are less organisms or when these are of a lower virulence. In certain diseases only chronic lesions are formed, for example in tuberculosis and syphilis.

Microscopically the lesion is less vascular, with few of the highly phagocytic polymorphs, but with more macrophages. If fibroblast activity is very intense many collagen fibres are laid down, and this leads to scarring. In this case resolution is impossible.

GENERAL REACTIONS TO INFECTION

Pathogenic organisms may exert their effects far away from the original site of infection, possibly leading to a general malaise, leucocytosis, and fever. There may be rigor, headache vomiting, raised temperature and pulse-rate.

Leucocytosis: Generalized increase of some or all of white blood-cells.

Rigor: Uncontrollable shivering.

TUBERCULOSIS

Chronic inflammatory condition due to *Mycobacterium tuberculosis*. This organism is very resistant to drying and may lie dormant in room dust. It can attack any organ, especially in people who are undernourished.

It usually enters the body via the nose or mouth as a droplet infection. From the mouth it may travel via the tonsils and lymphatics to the cervical lymph-glands, which themselves become infected. Nasal infections tend to affect the lungs and their lymph-glands.

OSTEOMYELITIS

Acute or chronic inflammation of bone. It may be caused by direct infection or by spread from the surrounding tissues. In the jaws, developing teeth may not form or may be deformed.

SYPHILIS

A chronic infective condition due to *Treponema pallidum*, a spiro-chaetal bacterium. As it cannot survive drying and dies outside the body, infection is only passed on by direct contact. Therefore dental surgeons take the precaution of wearing rubber gloves whilst operating in the mouths of syphilitic patients.

Syphilis in a pregnant woman can lead to infection of the foetus, which may be born dead, die soon, or bear a variety of lesions.

TETANUS

A serious disease due to *Clostridium tetani*, a spore-forming bacillus. It produces an extremely potent toxin, and is therefore highly dangerous. The spores can withstand boiling for up to an hour and can survive drying for months. They are widely distributed in dust and cause disease when taken with dirt into wounds. As the organism is anaerobic it grows and multiplies in fairly deep wounds, away from oxygen.

The bacillus tends to remain at the site of entry, but it releases toxins which attack the nervous system. This may lead to spasm or contraction of muscles supplied by the diseased nerve. One of the earliest manifestations may be lock-jaw (contraction of the masseter muscles). Other muscles are affected later. The patient finally dies of heart failure, asphyxia, or secondary infection.

DISTURBANCES OF CIRCULATION
Clotting

Physiological stoppage of bleeding by formation of a fibrin network which traps red blood-cells and platelets. Normal clotting time is about 4 minutes. Clotting is delayed where there is a deficiency of fibrin, platelets, or anti-haemophilic globulin.

Haemophilia

A disturbance of clotting due to lack of anti-haemophilic globulin in the blood. It is a sex-linked hereditary disease which only occurs in males. Although females do not show symptoms, they may pass it on to their male children.

Because of the greatly prolonged bleeding period careful precautions must be taken prior to operations or patients may bleed to death. For dental extractions:—

1. The patient is admitted to hospital.
2. Impressions are taken beforehand and a splint is constructed. After tooth extraction the splint is cemented on to the remaining teeth.

It protects the clot and helps to prevent bleeding by applying pressure.

3. A transfusion of plasma containing anti-haemophilic globulin is given to aid clotting.

4. If possible, sutures are not used as these will themselves cause bleeding.

5. For a similar reason injections are avoided.

As it is best to avoid extractions at all costs, such patients should attend regularly for routine dental care.

Thrombosis

Pathological clotting within blood-vessels, thereby blocking further passage of blood. Although this causes the patient a certain amount of distress, that part of the body receiving its blood via this vessel will usually tend to receive an increased supply of blood from elsewhere, recovery therefore taking place. However, as heart-muscle is not well supplied by alternative vessels, thrombosis of a coronary artery leads to permanent damage of the area supplied. Part of the thrombus may become detached from the main lesion and be carried around in the blood-stream as an embolus.

Emboli

Foreign bodies of various kinds which are carried around in the blood-stream. They eventually become impacted and prevent blood passing that point.

a. Thrombus: Embolus of blood-clot.

b. Air: May enter via a cut artery. In the heart it interferes with the passage of blood, rapidly leading to death.

c. Fat: This can enter the blood-stream from a damaged bone.

Atheroma

A degenerative condition affecting arteries. Projections into the lumen of vessels slow down the passage of blood. The surface of these projections becomes roughened and causes thrombosis to occur at that point.

Haemorrhage

Loss of blood from a vessel. Prolonged bleeding may be due to initial lack of clotting (primary haemorrhage) or later disturbance of a formed clot (secondary haemorrhage).

GENERAL CAUSES

Stoppage of bleeding is slower in people with haemorrhagic conditions such as haemophilia and purpura.

LOCAL CAUSES

Damage to a main artery or many small vessels provides little protection for the clot, allowing its mechanical displacement.

The above general (systemic) and local factors contribute to primary haemorrhage. Secondary haemorrhage occurs when a formed clot is disturbed by trauma. For example, biting a crust of bread may displace a clot. Tertiary haemorrhage occurs when a clot becomes infected and broken down, bleeding then recurring.

NECROSIS

Death of cells and tissues. It may be caused by trauma, chemical, bacterial, and physical agents, and loss of blood-supply. Thus blockage of a coronary artery by an embolus leads to degeneration and necrosis of cardiac muscle.

Gangrene

Necrosis plus infection by putrefactive micro-organisms, which thrive upon dead cells. Gangrene is divided clinically into dry, moist, and gaseous varieties. Gas gangrene occurs after infection by the bacterium *Clostridium welchii*. These are anaerobic and thus flourish and produce gas in the depths of wounds, especially in muscle. It is therefore essential to cleanse such wounds carefully after accidents.

HYPERTROPHY, HYPERPLASIA, AND ATROPHY

Hypertrophy: Increase in size of a tissue or organ due to enlargement of the individual cells.

Hyperplasia: Increased size due to an increased *number* of cells, not to their enlargement.

Atrophy: Reduced size of a tissue or organ due to a reduction in size of individual cells.

Hypertrophy and hyperplasia may occur together, and can be due to physiological and pathological causes. In trained athletes the heart ventricular muscle often hypertrophies in response to increased demands. In pregnancy the uterus undergoes hypertrophic enlargement. Compensatory hypertrophy may occur in the remaining organ when one of a pair has been removed, for example after loss of a diseased kidney.

Physiological hyperplasia of red blood-cells occurs as a response to the prolonged anoxia experienced at high altitudes. Mountain climbers may spend several days at each stage of ascent to allow their blood to adapt to the decreased atmospheric oxygen. As each cell receives less oxygen the body compensates by a hyperplastic increase in the number of red blood-cells. Thus the total amount of circulating oxygen remains constant.

Pathological hyperplasia occurs following a single severe haemorrhage, with loss of many red cells. Irritation by a poorly fitting denture may cause a hyperplastic overgrowth of oral mucosa around the denture periphery.

Atrophy occurs as a physiological response to disuse of a part. After extraction of a tooth the alveolar bone is no longer needed to form a socket, so it is resorbed and the overlying gum shrinks. When limbs are immobilized in the treatment of fractures their muscles often visibly atrophy. They are therefore exercised by physiotherapists. Constant pressure may also cause atrophy. This is useful to orthodontists. Pressure from springs causes teeth to press on bone, making the latter resorb. The teeth then move into the space vacated.

Cardiac-muscle cells atrophy when their blood-supply is slowly decreased, for example during pathological narrowing of the arteries by atheroma formation.

NEOPLASIA

Formation of a new growth or tumour.

Tumour

Abnormal mass of tissue growing at an abnormal rate, which continues to grow after the removal of the original stimulus. It thus differs from a hyperplastic response which stops with removal of the stimulus and may even be reversed. Tumours are benign or malignant.

BENIGN

Slow-growing, harmless, and tend to be confined to the area of origin.

MALIGNANT

Fast-growing tumours that may spread to other parts of the body, resulting in widespread damage and often causing death.

GENERAL REACTIONS TO TRAUMA

Earlier in the chapter we discussed the localized responses of inflammation. With a more severe stimulus, or in a very sensitive person, there may be a generalized effect away from the site of damage. This is based on the physiological response to alarm, fear, or rage.

Shock

Clinical condition resulting from a severe reduction in volume and pressure of the circulating blood. It is divided into primary and secondary varieties.

PRIMARY

Occurs immediately or within a few hours of application of the stimulus. The patient is pale, cold, and sweating. He may appear apathetic, or listless and frightened. Nausea, vomiting, and fainting sometimes occur. The patient should be made to lie down, and is kept warm with a blanket.

SECONDARY

This is much more serious. It may develop several hours after the primary shock, and is often associated with severe blood or fluid loss. It may thus follow severe burning. The patient appears weak, listless, and depressed. His pulse is rapid and feeble, and the temperature low. Respiration is rapid and shallow. The hands and feet feel very cold and the face is pale and moist, with the eyes sunken. The patient is often thirsty, but may vomit if given a drink. Such patients should be immediately transferred to hospital, where a blood transfusion will probably be given.

BURNS AND SCALDS

Burns: Injuries caused by heat, electric currents, X-rays, and ultra-violet light. They vary considerably, from slight hyperaemia and reddening of the surface skin to massive necrosis of the deepest layers.

Scalds: Burns due to moist heat, such as boiling water.

Burns and scalds are extremely painful, and may be accompanied by shock, infection, persistent ulceration, and deformity. These may be minimized by adequate and immediate treatment.

TREATMENT OF BURNS AND SCALDS

1. Removal of the cause.
2. Prevention and treatment of shock.
3. Prevention of sepsis by cleansing the area with a detergent such as Cetavlon, and applying a gauze dressing. An antibiotic may be administered systemically if there is severe wounding.
4. Promotion of healing and prevention of deformity. In very deep burns a skin-graft may be needed. Once such a graft has taken, gentle exercises are started to prevent contraction of the area.

Chemical Injuries

Corrosive chemicals such as strong acids and alkalis can seriously damage skin and mucosa, producing lesions closely resembling burns. The immediate treatment is to rapidly neutralize and wash off the irritant.

Burnt or Scalded Mouths

Such injuries may be caused by extremely hot fluids, corrosive poisons, or, in the case of small children, by putting their mouths to the spout of a hot kettle. There is a danger that swelling of the oral tissues may make it difficult to breathe.

TREATMENT

1. If the patient is conscious give cold water to drink or ice to suck.
2. If unconscious, lie him on his back, with his head on the side.
3. Ensure that he can breathe.
4. If necessary, give artificial respiration.
5. Send for an ambulance.

QUESTIONS

1. Describe the expected appearance of inflamed skin or mucosa.
2. Discuss the causes of bleeding.
3. What are:—
    a. Hyperplasia ?
    b. Hypertrophy ?
    c. Atrophy ?
4. Discuss the causes and treatment of shock.

CHAPTER VI

ORAL PATHOLOGY

DENTAL CARIES

DISEASE of the hard tissues of the teeth leading to loss of inorganic (hard) constituents and eventual disintegration of the organic matrix. As with all pathological processes we must understand the nature of the causative factors before we are able to prevent the disease. Disease occurs when the attacking factors are stronger than the defensive ones.

Attack	*Defence*
Micro-organisms	Tooth shape (morphology)
Bacterial plaque	Tooth structure
Refined carbohydrates	Tooth position
	Muscular action
	Saliva
	Oral hygiene

Attack

The main factors of attack to be considered are micro-organisms, plaque, and refined carbohydrates (*Fig.* 29).

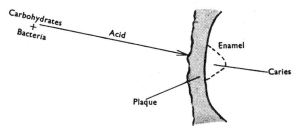

Fig. 29.—Attack on tooth enamel by acids formed from carbohydrates by bacteria. Caries develops below the acid-retaining plaque.

MICRO-ORGANISMS

Many are normally present in the oral cavity. Acidogenic bacteria, such as lactobacilli, act on refined carbohydrates to break them down, first to simple sugars and then to acids. The latter initiate the carious process by dissolving out mineral salts from enamel. The number of lactobacilli present in a mouth tends to be directly proportional to the intake of refined carbohydrates. This forms the basis of the lactobacillus count, in which the dentist checks the carbohydrate intake of his patient by counting the lactobacilli present in the mouth.

Other bacteria release proteolytic enzymes, which act on the remaining organic substance to cause the final breakdown of tooth structure. The carious process in dentine is very similar to that in enamel, but progresses more quickly.

BACTERIAL PLAQUE

This forms a layer on the surface of teeth. It consists of thread-like organisms, cocci, bacilli, mucin, epithelial debris, food remnants, and any other substances that collect in the mouth. It tends to gather more readily in stagnation areas, where it holds acids in contact with the tooth surface, thus prolonging the period of enamel attack and breakdown. It is therefore advantageous to remove such plaque by regular prophylaxis of the teeth.

REFINED CARBOHYDRATES

By 'refinement' we mean the treatment of flour, sugar, and other carbohydrates in order to make them whiter, to remove any fibrous material, and to adjust their taste. The refinement of cereal and flour leads to a smaller grain size, with less fibrous elements. Refined carbohydrates quickly become sticky and cling to the tooth surface. As they are easily broken down to form acids they should be excluded from the diet. The total quantity of calories for energy may be made up by eating more meat, eggs, milk, and vegetables.

Defensive Factors

Under this heading we include morphology, structure and position of teeth, muscular action, saliva, and oral hygiene methods. The latter will be considered in Chapter XV.

TOOTH MORPHOLOGY (SHAPE)

Caries occurs more readily in stagnation areas, for example, in anatomical pits and fissures, at hypoplastic defects, and below contact points. It is thus more commonly found in molars and premolars than in incisors and canines. However, deep pits are sometimes seen on the palatal surfaces of upper lateral incisors.

TOOTH STRUCTURE

Caries occurs less easily, and therefore more slowly, in a well calcified tooth. An even greater resistance to the dissolving of enamel by acids, is conferred by the presence of a substantial amount of fluoride in the surface layer of enamel. The fluoride content can be slightly increased after tooth eruption, but for maximum effect should be introduced in water during tooth formation. Thus nutrition is of the utmost importance at that time. The diet must include adequate supplies of vitamins A, C, and D, calcium, phosphorus, and fluoride. Apart from nutritional factors, the resistance of teeth to decay is partly determined by hereditary or genetic factors (family background).

Tooth Position

Abnormally placed teeth prevent adequate natural and artificial cleansing and therefore lead to stagnation. This includes rotated, tilted, instanding, and bucally placed teeth. It is important to avoid extractions as loss of a single tooth leads to undesirable movements of those teeth remaining around the gap. Malpositioned teeth should be corrected by early orthodontic therapy.

Muscular Action

Constant action of tongue, lips, and cheek muscles cleanses accessible tooth surfaces by friction. However, this is not always possible in spastics and patients suffering from certain conditions of muscular paralysis.

Saliva

Watery saliva washes food debris away from teeth whereas sticky viscous saliva aids its retention. Salivary flow decreases during feverish illnesses, so increased attention should be paid to artificial mouth cleansing at such times. Saliva tends to dilute and neutralize any acid products present in the oral cavity. In addition it has antibacterial action due to the presence of certain enzymes.

Sites of Onset of Caries

Caries can commence in various positions, cavities being classified according to site of onset.

Class I

Begin in anatomical pits and fissures. It thus usually refers to cavities in molars and premolars, but palatal pits in upper lateral incisors are included.

Class II

Onset is between the teeth, in the interproximal regions of molars and premolars.

CLASS III

Start interproximally, between anterior teeth.

CLASS IV

Interproximal caries of anterior teeth involving the incisal surface.

CLASS V

Cavities beginning in the gingival third of buccal and lingual surfaces.

Colour of Caries

The initial caries lesion is white. Although fast-spreading decay tends to retain this colour, the slower varieties become stained and appear brown. Secondary caries looks bluish-white when seen through the surface enamel.

Spread

The lesion spreads from the outer enamel surface towards the dentine. It is funnel-shaped, with the widest part towards the outside. At the

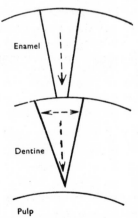

Fig. 30.—Arrow shows direction of spread of caries through enamel and dentine.

amelodentinal junction between enamel and dentine, it suddenly spreads sideways. From there it again spreads funnel-like through the dentine, towards the pulp. The final microscopic appearance is therefore rather like one funnel balanced upon another (*Fig.* 30). Secondary caries may spread from the amelodentinal junction back towards the enamel surface, through which it is seen as a bluish-white discoloration.

Sequelae

Untreated caries usually leads to hyperaemia, pulpitis, death of the pulp, and finally abscess formation. Occasionally the process is arrested.

Arrested Caries

If caries is removed from the tooth and the initiating factor eliminated, no further damage will usually occur. Sometimes the destructive process halts spontaneously, the lesion becoming dark brown and very hard. This is known as arrested caries. It is due to the elimination of food-retaining areas such as jagged enamel surfaces. Such areas may break away during mastication, but arrest can be induced in the surgery by the dentist grinding them away. Acid-producing foods are therefore no longer retained in contact with the tooth, and the carious process stops.

HYPERAEMIA AND PULPITIS

When the carious process is allowed to continue, it progresses through the dentine towards the pulp. This irritates odontoblast fibres in the dentine and causes inflammation in the pulp itself. The initial inflammatory response is 'hyperaemia' (increased blood-flow). If the irritant is removed at this stage the reaction may cease and may even be reversed with the pulp reverting to its original state. Otherwise it progresses to a state of 'pulpitis', which is a more acute and irreversible inflammatory condition.

Aetiology of Pulpitis

1. Caries.
2. Acid-containing filling materials placed in deep cavities. It is thus essential to place a lining below silicates and similar filling materials.
3. A severe bang on a tooth, for example during hockey or netball, irrespective of whether or not the pulp is exposed.
4. Overheating the tooth during cavity preparation. Tooth and bur should therefore be cooled with water.

DENTAL ABSCESS

With severe inflammation the pulp swells. As it is contained within a firm tooth structure, it tends to constrict itself, and cuts off its own blood-supply. This results in death and degeneration of the pulp, and then abscess formation. The pulpal abscess spreads out of the tooth to involve *first* the supporting tissues (apical abscess) and then the surrounding bone (alveolar abscess). Finally, pus may drain from the bone into the mouth, via a sinus (*Fig.* 31).

Any abscess may be acute or chronic. The acute form is characterized by an intense throbbing pain, whereas the chronic type is dull and nagging in nature, and may be hardly noticed by the patient.

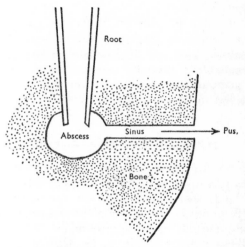

Fig. 31.—Spread of pus from apical abscess.

ATTRITION

Wearing away of tooth cusps of teeth during chewing movements. It occurs very slowly in most adults, but more quickly in the deciduous dentition. Gross attrition occurs:—

1. In spastics, who exhibit continual grinding movements.

2. In otherwise normal people who grind their teeth during the night (bruxism). Less food tends to be retained on these teeth, with a subsequent decrease in caries. In most cases attrition tends to be painless.

ABRASION

Wearing away of tooth enamel due to *external* agents. Thus, incorrect use of a toothbrush with horizontal instead of vertical movements tends to abrade the cervical margin enamel, especially in teeth standing out from the arch. It has also been caused by holding hard objects such as pins and nails between the teeth, habits practised by hairdressers, upholsterers, cobblers, and many other tradespeople. Eventually the sensitive dentine layer is exposed, and there is discomfort from heat, cold, sweet, sour, and brushing. This pain is usually transient and goes away. Sometimes sodium fluoride paste is applied as an obtundent. If the discomfort is excessive a filling may be placed.

EROSION

Rarer than abrasion and attrition, this refers to loss of tooth substance by dissolving agencies. It may occur in factory workers exposed to certain chemicals, for example, those involved in the manufacture of car batteries, and also with excessive consumption of lemon juice and undiluted iron medicines and vitamin syrups.

DISCOLORATION OF TEETH

Stains may be extrinsic or intrinsic.

1. Extrinsic (on the outside of the enamel)

Occur more frequently in the presence of roughened enamel, irregular teeth, decreased mastication, sticky saliva, gingival pockets and other stagnation areas, and poor oral hygiene.

a. CALCULUS

Calculus or tartar consists of mineral salts such as calcium phosphate, with some carbonate, fluoride, and magnesium phosphate. These are embedded in a network of filamentous bacteria, desquamated epithelial cells, blood cells, and other debris, the whole mass being attached to the tooth surface. Calculus may be sub- or supragingival.

i. *Supragingival:* Above gum level, especially on tooth surfaces opposite salivary gland ducts; thus lingual to lower incisors, buccal to upper molars. It is less common in children. The light brown colour darkens in the presence of tobacco and some foods.

ii. *Subgingival:* Below the gingival margin it is more firmly adherent, as it contacts rougher cementum. It is usually brownish-green, but being stained mostly with blood products their breakdown can lead to a variety of colours.

b. GREEN STAIN

Probably due to remnants of Nasmyth's membrane (combined outer and inner enamel epithelium) which is later stained by chromogenic or pigment-producing bacteria. It usually occurs in the cervical third of teeth in patients with poor oral hygiene. As it tends to act as a site for decalcification and decay it must be removed with a stiff bristle brush and pumice.

c. BLACK LINES

More commonly found in children, even in relatively clean mouths. They usually occur close to the gingival margins especially on the palatal surface, and tend to be associated with a low caries rate.

d. BLACK OR DARK BROWN AREAS

Patients using stannous fluoride toothpastes sometimes exhibit dark brown or black stains in the cervical area of enamel. They may be regarded as evidence of poor oral hygiene resulting in retention of materia alba, which becomes stained. It may be prevented by improved toothbrushing techniques.

2. Intrinsic (forms part of the structure)

a. CARIES

Early decalcified areas are white, but they take up oral stains and become brown. Rapidly spreading decay has less chance to absorb stains and so it is lighter in colour.

Secondary caries is that which has spread internally from another part of the tooth and therefore has no contact with the external surface. It appears to be pale blue in colour when viewed through the enamel.

b. BLOOD-BORNE PIGMENTS

In haemolytic disease of the newborn red blood-cells are broken down and bile is released. This may become incorporated into the structure of deciduous teeth to give them a blue-green or yellow colour.

c. TETRACYCLINE STAINING

It is sometimes necessary to administer one of the tetracycline antibiotic drugs to combat infection. If taken during the period of tooth formation it may be incorporated into its structure, appearing clinically as a yellow discoloration of the tooth.

d. NON-VITAL TEETH

With death of the pulp, blood-cells present in the pulp chamber disintegrate and release haemoglobin. This in turn is broken down to form various pigments which stain the dentine and give the tooth a darkened appearance. The discoloration is similar to a bruise.

ANOMALIES OF TEETH

1. Missing.
2. Supernumeraries (additional teeth).
3. Malformations—including peg-shaped teeth, hypocalcification, hypoplasia.

Hypoplastic Teeth

Hypoplasia is a cellular or structural defect of enamel characterized by pits, lines, and other deficiencies. It is caused by damage to the ameloblasts whilst these are forming the enamel matrix.

Hypocalcified Teeth

A defect due to damage during the calcifying stage. It therefore results not in deficiency of tissue, but in enamel that is softer than usual.

Both conditions may be due to systemic and localized disturbances. Some childhood fevers affect the development of all teeth forming at that time, resulting in either hypoplasia or hypocalcification according to the developmental stage reached. Localized infections affect individual teeth forming in that area. Thus a root abscess on a deciduous incisor may affect the colour of its permanent successor.

Amelogenesis Imperfecta

Hereditary condition of poorly developed enamel, resulting in hypoplasia or hypocalcification of many teeth. This poses a problem of aesthetics, and usually necessitates the placing of many crowns.

Dentinogenesis Imperfecta

Hereditary defect of teeth resulting in a brown opalescent appearance and brittle enamel.

CHRONIC MARGINAL GINGIVITIS

A slowly progressive inflammation of gingival tissues, usually resulting from poor oral hygiene. Debris and other material stagnate in areas where tooth cleansing is inadequate, such as around poorly fitting partial dentures and orthodontic appliances, and edges on fillings. Bacteria grow and multiply in such sites, causing gingival inflammation. Calculus also readily gives rise to irritation. Prolonged mouth breathing causes drying of the oral tissues, inadequate natural cleansing of gingivae, and eventually gingivitis.

CLINICAL FEATURES

The gums become redder, swollen and shiny. Unfortunately this swelling itself provides deep (false) pockets in which more food debris may stagnate (*Fig.* 32). The gingivae bleed easily with the slightest touch, making patients afraid to brush their teeth and gums, this in

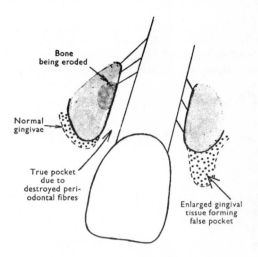

Fig. 32.—Diagram of periodontal disease.

turn leading to a worsening of the condition. In fact the correct treatment would be to brush the gums more frequently. Brushing plus chewing of hard fibrous foods hardens the surface gingival layer, which makes it more resistant to further attack, and also removes food and other irritants.

ACUTE ULCERATIVE GINGIVITIS (VINCENT'S DISEASE)

The onset is usually rapid, the patient complaining of severe pain, gums that bleed readily, and bad breath. It is often superimposed on a previously present chronic marginal gingivitis. The mouth is usually dirty, with debris and calculus around the teeth. The gingivae are red, swollen, and tender, and bleed with the slight touch. The interdental papillae become ulcerated.

In severe cases the patient feels unwell, with fever and enlarged lymph-glands. The condition may be contagious. Organisms such as the spiral-shaped *Treponema vincenti* and the spindle-shaped *Bacillus fusiformis* have been shown to be present in the mouths of such patients.

PREGNANCY GINGIVITIS

The gingivae sometimes become swollen and inflamed at this time, and occasionally give rise to a small enlargement known as a ' pregnancy tumour '. The cause is probably hormonal. It is essential to practise a high standard of oral hygiene to prevent local irritation making this condition worse.

EPANUTIN HYPERPLASTIC GINGIVAE

An overgrowth of the gingivae sometimes occurs in epileptics taking the drug Epanutin or Dilantin Sodium (phenytoin). It may reach as far as the incisal margins of the teeth.

CHRONIC PERIODONTITIS

A slowly progressing inflammatory lesion of the dental supporting structures, it is the main cause of loss of teeth in later adult life. Chronic periodontitis follows from untreated chronic gingivitis. Progressive infection and inflammation gradually destroy periodontal membrane and surrounding bone, creating deep (true) pockets in which further irritants lodge and bacteria multiply (*see Fig.* 32). Eventually there is a purulent discharge, foul taste, and gross loosening of the teeth.

LATERAL PARODONTAL ABSCESS

Highly infective organisms in the periodontal membrane cause gross inflammatory changes, breakdown of the membrane, and pus formation. Bacteria may enter via a deep pathological pocket or through a hole made traumatically, for example, by a fishbone.

The gums are very sore and painful, with pus exuding from a pocket. A sinus may point into the buccal sulcus. Although the related tooth may be tender to touch it remains vital, thus being differentiated from an apical abscess.

PERICORONITIS

Food and bacteria accumulate below gum flaps around erupting teeth, especially around the mandibular wisdom teeth. With inflammation the flap swells and contacts the occluding tooth, from which trauma causes further inflammation and swelling.

Clinically the flap is seen to be swollen and possibly ulcerated. Much pain may radiate to the teeth and ear. Halitosis and a foul taste may be present and the patient may not be able to open his mouth fully. This latter condition is called 'trismus'. In severe cases the regional lymph-glands may be enlarged.

HERPETIC STOMATITIS

A fairly common condition caused by the herpes simplex virus. Initial infection usually takes place at some time during the first six years of life. Although usually mild, it occasionally takes the form of an acute stomatitis. In such cases there are often many painful ulcers in a very sore mouth, making it extremely difficult to eat anything other than ice-cream or jelly. In addition the regional lymph-glands enlarge, there may be a high temperature, and the child feels generally unwell. It usually takes between seven and ten days before recovery takes place.

After the primary infection patients tend to go through life with recurrent but much milder attacks. These may take the form of cold sores on the lips.

APHTHOUS ULCERS

Very painful ulcers which occur in the mouths of some patients at regular intervals. The exact cause is unknown, but they may be associated with stomach upsets, hormonal disturbances, or allergies. Many people get them when feeling run down or worried, such as at examination time. The painful phase tends to disappear after about four days.

DRY SOCKET

Infected socket, usually following loss of its blood-clot. The bone becomes exposed, inflamed, and very painful.

QUESTIONS

1. A girl aged 13 has developed a large number of carious cavities over the past year:—
   a. For what reasons may this have occurred ?
   b. What advice may be given to the patient ?
   c. How may these carious cavities be detected and treated in their earliest stages ?
2. What is acute ulcerative gingivitis (Vincent's infection) and what particular precautions are necessary in the dental surgery in connexion with this condition ?
3. Discuss the cause and results of a dental abscess.
4. Describe and discuss plaque.

CHAPTER VII

MICROBIOLOGY AND THE PRINCIPLES OF STERILIZATION

MICROBIOLOGY

THE study of living organisms which can only be seen through a microscope. These include bacteria, fungi, viruses, and protozoa. As some cause disease it is important to know something of their life history in order to prevent their growth and multiplication.

The first person to see and describe micro-organisms was van Leeuwenhoek, a Dutchman living in the seventeenth century. His microscope consisted of a single small magnifying glass held in a metal frame. In 1683 he examined water from pools and fæces from a case of dysentery, and was amazed to see what he called tiny 'animalcules'. Later, scientists began to associate microscopic organisms with the causation of certain diseases.

CLASSIFICATION OF MICRO-ORGANISMS

1. *Bacteria:* Includes main group of disease-causing organisms.

2. *Fungi:* Yeasts and moulds, such as seen on damp stale bread.

3. *Viruses:* Organisms too small to be seen with the normal microscope.

4. *Protozoa:* Microscopic animals including amoebae and malarial parasites.

5. *Rickettsiae:* Bacteria-like organisms probably belonging to the vegetable kingdom. They cause diseases such as Rocky Mountain spotted fever.

6. *Algae:* Green plants including seaweeds.

Apart from the algae all these groups contain some organisms which are pathogenic or disease-producing. This word is derived from the Greek 'patho' meaning sadness or pain, and 'genic' meaning to produce or cause. For our present purposes we will only consider bacteria, fungi, and viruses.

Bacteria

Very small organisms which can only be seen with a microscope. They are divided into sub-groups according to their morphology and arrangement (*Fig.* 33).

1. COCCI (round cells):—
    a. Staphylococci (in clusters): Found in boils, carbuncles and similar lesions.

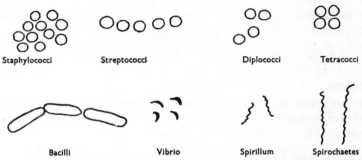

| Staphylococci | Streptococci | Diplococci | Tetracocci |

| Bacilli | Vibrio | Spirillum | Spirochaetes |

Fig. 33.—Some typical shapes and arrangements of micro-organisms.

   b. Streptococci (in chains): Causative organisms of scarlet fever, tonsillitis, and rheumatic fever.
   c. Diplococci (in pairs): *Diplococcus pneumoniæ* causes pneumonia.
   d. Tetracocci (in groups of four): Found in dental and pulmonary abscesses, and cervical adenitis.
   e. Sarcinae (cuboidal groups of eight).
2. BACILLI (straight, rod-shaped cylinders):—
    E.g., *Corynebacterium diphtheriae*, the causative organism of diphtheria; *Mycobacterium tuberculosis*, the causative organism of tuberculosis; *Clostridium tetani*, the causative organism of tetanus; *Clostridium welchii*, the causative organism of gas gangrene.
3. VIBRIO (curved but rigid bacilli).
4. SPIRILLA (wavy but rigid bacilli).
5. SPIROCHAETES (long and thin, spirally coiled, capable of flexing and twisting movements):—
    E.g., *Treponema pallidum*, the causative organism of syphilis; *Treponema vincenti*, the causative organism of acute ulcerative gingivitis.
6. LEPTOTHRIX (unbranched filamentous organisms).
7. STREPTOTHRIX (branched filamentous organisms):—
    E.g., *Actinomyces israeli*, which causes actinomycosis.
    The pathological features of the more important examples of the above groups are referred to in the next chapter.

BACTERIAL SPORES

Some bacteria form a hard, thick-walled membrane or spore as a reaction to adverse environmental conditions. This can withstand chemical and physical agents that normally destroy the usual vegetative or sporeless forms. Some may resist boiling for up to an hour and drying for very long periods. They may persist in dust and soil for years, and then germinate in more favourable conditions. It is therefore most important to know which organisms produce spores, and how they may be destroyed. It is also essential to ensure that no dust is allowed to remain in surgical areas. Amongst the spore-forming organisms are those causing anthrax, tetanus, and food poisoning.

CAPSULES

Some bacteria produce a slimy coating or capsule which makes them very resistant to attack by white blood-cells and other body defences. They are therefore highly infective.

RESPIRATION OR BREATHING

All bacteria need oxygen in order to live and multiply.

1. *Aerobes:* Derive oxygen directly from the air.

2. *Anaerobes:* Gain their oxygen by the breakdown of proteins and carbohydrates, but are inhibited by the presence of free oxygen.

3. *Facultative anaerobes:* Normally live in the presence of free oxygen, but can survive under anaerobic conditions.

Fungi

The study of fungi, which are primitive forms of plant life devoid of chlorophyll, is known as mycology. There is much variation in the size of fungi, from the microscopic yeasts to the large mushrooms and toadstools. The moulds and yeasts are of medical importance.

MOULDS

Multicellular organisms with their cells lying end to end to form long filaments or hyphae. These gather together to form mouldy patches, such as may be seen on bread and meat. A very important mould is *Penicillium notatum*, from which penicillin is produced.

YEASTS

Unicellular fungi which occur naturally in grapes and other fruits, playing a part in the fermentation processes involved in the manufacture of wines, beer, and bread.

Candida albicans is a yeast responsible for the disease moniliasis or thrush. This occurs in bottle-fed infants, and also beneath dentures and orthodontic appliances.

Viruses

Minute organisms smaller than bacteria, which cannot be cultivated outside living cells, can only be seen with an electron (very powerful) microscope, and which can pass through minute filters that prevent the passage of bacteria and fungi. Viruses may be spherical, rod-shaped, or cuboidal. They cause such diseases as the common cold, influenza, poliomyelitis, mumps, measles, chicken pox, and acute infective hepatitis.

Viruses are resistant to most types of sterilization and to antibiotics, but dry heat and autoclave sterilizers effectively destroy them.

INFECTION

Invasion of tissues by micro-organisms and the damage caused by their establishment and multiplication. It results in an inflammatory reaction, in a similar way to that caused by physical and chemical agents. The resultant tissue changes were dealt with in Chapter V. The degree of subsequent damage depends upon the number and virulence of the organisms, and on the resistance of the host. Some viruses rapidly gain in strength as they pass from one host to another.

Spread of Infection

a. In some cases the causative organism may already be present in the body. For example, most infections of the dental pulp are due to organisms normally present in the mouth.

b. Infection may be passed on by a person suffering from the disease.

c. Sometimes the source of infection is a 'carrier', a person who carries the organisms but who does not himself show clinical manifestations of the disease.

In order to prevent the spread of infection, it is essential to understand the means by which organisms pass from person to person. They are transmitted in one or more of the following ways:—

1. DIRECT CONTACT

Diseases such as syphilis are caused by organisms which tend not to survive outside the body. Therefore infecting organisms are passed on by direct contact, sexual or otherwise.

2. DROPLET INFECTION

The causative organisms of respiratory infections are sprayed from the body during bouts of coughing and sneezing, and are carried around in the atmosphere before reaching a new host.

3. TRANSMISSION BY INSECTS

In some diseases the organisms are carried from person to person by means of insect carriers. Thus the malarial parasite is carried between humans by means of mosquitoes.

4. OTHER VEHICLES

Infecting organisms such as those causing tuberculosis and typhoid are carried in milk and water. Intestinal organisms can be passed on by people who do not wash their hands after going to the lavatory.

ENTRY OF ORGANISMS TO A NEW HOST

1. Via skin and mucous membranes, possibly through cuts, small abrasions, and bites. The infective hepatitis virus can be transmitted by non-sterile needles.

2. Through the mouth during ingestion of food.

3. Via the nose during respiration.

Resistance against Infection

1. *Skin secretions:* These possess certain fatty acids with anti-bacterial action.

2. *Desquamation of skin epithelial cells:* Surface cells are continually being shed, taking with them any adherent organisms. Cells from the oral mucosa are swallowed.

3. *Saliva:* This contains enzymes that are slightly bactericidal against those bacteria not normally found in the mouth. In addition the fluid washes out the oral cavity, this aiding the removal of micro-organisms.

4. *Cilia in the respiratory tract:* Tiny hairlike structures trap debris and organisms, and prevent their passage down the respiratory tract into the lungs. Movement of these cilia tends to return the entrapped substances to the pharynx.

5. *Immunity.*

STERILIZATION

This is a process that renders a contaminated object sterile or free from micro-organisms, including viruses and bacterial spores. Both physical and chemical methods are used. The technique chosen depends partly upon the material to be sterilized, so that it is not damaged in any way.

Physical Methods

1. DRY HEAT

   a. Exposure to a naked flame: The very high temperature of a flame rapidly kills organisms. Apart from laboratory use this method has few other applications.

   b. Hot-air ovens: Even resistant spores are killed if exposed to 160° C. for 45 minutes. At higher temperatures items such as paper points are damaged. For metals, 18 minutes at 170° C., and 7½ minutes at 180° C. are equally effective. These temperatures must be maintained, so sterilizer doors must remain closed. Instruments should first be washed and *dried*.

   c. Heated salt and glass beads: These are heated electrically or by means of a burner to maintain a very high temperatured environment into which instruments can be dipped. They are very useful for root-canal instruments.

2. MOIST HEAT

   a. Boiling water: Instruments must be scrubbed clean and then boiled for at least 20 minutes at 100° C. During this time no other instruments must be added. Boiling sterilizers are tending to be replaced by autoclaves and hot-air ovens, as spores are not killed by this method.

   b. The autoclave: Water is boiled under pressure. Even the most resistant spores are killed after 15 minutes exposure at 120° C., or 10 minutes at 126° C.

3. IRRADIATION

   Certain objects such as hypodermic needles and surgical gloves are sterilized by exposure to gamma rays. These materials should be disposed of after use if the full advantages of sterility are to be maintained.

Chemical Methods

Before considering these it is useful to define some terms.

Bactericide: Any agent that kills bacteria.

Bacteriostat: An agent that prevents growth and multiplication of bacteria without actually killing them. It gives the body's natural defences a chance to kill off the organisms.

Disinfectants: Bactericidal preparations of such high concentrations that they must not come into contact with the skin or mucosa. They are used to decontaminate instruments in the laboratory.

Antiseptics: These are weaker so can be brought into contact with the skin. They are used for the prevention and treatment of tissue infections.

For chemical agents to exert their maximum effect they must be brought into intimate contact with the object concerned. Therefore all debris, including blood and pus, must first be removed. A few chemical agents are considered below. They must be diluted as recommended by the manufacturers. *N.B.*, For a 5 per cent solution (1 in 20) use 1 part chemical, 19 of water.

1. SOAP AND WATER

In addition to the physical action of removing debris and organisms, some soaps are bacteriostatic.

2. 70 PER CENT ALCOHOL

As well as being itself bacteriostatic alcohol is used as a solvent for other antibacterial agents such as iodine.

3. IODINE

Aqueous solutions of iodine and potassium iodide are widely used. Alcoholic iodine solutions and tinctures are used as skin antiseptics.

4. HYDROGEN PEROXIDE

This gives off oxygen bubbles which mechanically dislodge debris and present an unfavourable environment for anaerobic organisms.

5. FORMALDEHYDE GAS

Given off by formalin tablets. Used to sterilize gutta-percha points. In aqueous solution it is known as 'formalin', which is widely used as a preserving agent for tissue specimens.

STERILIZATION IN DENTAL PRACTICE

For convenience this will be considered under four headings.
1. Sterilization of mucous membranes.
2. Sterilization of surgical instruments.
3. Sterilization for root-canal therapy.
4. Sterilization of other instruments.

1. Mucous Membranes

The mucosal surface is sterilized prior to any operation in order to prevent the transmission of organisms into the deeper tissues. Two per cent iodine in 70 per cent alcohol is often used.

2. Surgical Instruments

As these penetrate the mucosa the highest degree of sterility must be maintained. Syringes and needles are best sterilized in autoclaves. Many dental surgeons today use needles that have been pre-sterilized by gamma radiation. After use these are thrown away and a new needle is used for each patient, in order to avoid the risk of transfer of the blood-borne Hepatitis virus.

All extraction and other surgical instruments should be sterilized by autoclave or dry heat, and then allowed to cool under a sterile towel. If wanted quickly they can be cooled in a weak antiseptic solution. Before boiling cutting instruments they should be wrapped in lint in order to prevent damage to their cutting edges.

3. Instruments for Root-canal Therapy

These are often made up as a kit in a metal box container and then autoclaved or subjected to dry heat. Gutta percha points and other items destroyed by heat are sterilized by storing with paraform tablets in an airtight container, the tablets giving off paraformaldehyde gas.

4. Other Instruments

Conventional handpieces are autoclaved or boiled in special oil, which is later allowed to drain off. For high-speed handpieces the manufacturer's instructions should be followed *closely*. Burs are cleaned with a sterile brush, sterilized in a chemical disinfectant and washed prior to use. Other instruments should be boiled for 20 minutes and stored in a closed container with paraform tablets in order to retain their sterility.

CHEMOTHERAPEUTIC AGENTS

These are chemicals synthesized so as to be lethal to bacteria but harmless to the tissues, and which can therefore be injected into the body. They are usually selective in their action against specific organisms, for example:—

1. Salvarsan against *Treponema pallidum*, the causative organism of syphilis.

2. Sulphonamides against staphylococci, streptococci, pneumococci.

ANTIBIOTICS

These are antibacterial agents synthesized from biological substances. The most famous is penicillin, manufactured from *Penicillium notatum*. This is completely harmless to the tissues. Tetracycline is another example.

Penicillin

This antibiotic is effective against a large number of bacteria. It has been incorporated into solutions, ointments, creams, lozenges, and chewing gum. However, it now tends to be confined to medicines, tablets, and injection solutions.

IMMUNITY

Antibacterial power of the blood, giving increased resistance to a disease. Immunity is divided into inherent and acquired varieties.

Inherent Immunity

Resistance that is already present at birth. It is mostly due to genetic factors. For example, certain animals are never affected by diseases such as measles and chicken-pox to which man is very susceptible. Inherent immunity varies a great deal between individuals.

Acquired Immunity

Resistance built up after birth. It may be divided into two types, active and passive, each of which is subdivided into natural and artificial varieties.

ACTIVE IMMUNITY

Conferred by passing through an attack of the disease in question, when a supply of defence cells or antibodies is formed in the body.

Active Natural Immunity: In this case the person gets a disease in the usual way and produces his own antibodies. With diseases such as mumps and poliomyelitis, the acquired immunity is usually retained for life. However, other diseases such as the common cold may recur.

Active Artificial Immunity: Here immunity is deliberately stimulated by the artificial introduction into the body of organisms (vaccines) or their products (toxoids).

Vaccines: Preparations containing organisms so modified as to stimulate immunity without causing the disease itself. They may consist of bacteria killed by heat or chemicals, for example T.A.B. vaccine used to prevent typhoid and paratyphoid. In certain cases killed organisms will not stimulate immunity. Instead we use living organisms with artificially lowered virulence. An example is the B.C.G. vaccine used to prevent tuberculosis. Small-pox vaccine also falls into this category.

Toxoids: Chemically modified toxins, the poisonous products of bacteria.

Artificial immunity is not as long lasting as the natural variety. Thus, whereas an attack of typhoid fever gives life-long immunity, T.A.B. vaccination must be repeated at fixed intervals.

PASSIVE IMMUNITY

Here the resistance is obtained by receipt of ready-made antibodies from another source.

Passive Natural Immunity: Natural transfer of ready-made antibodies from another source. Thus, during pregnancy, the foetus obtains antibodies from its mother. Such immunity is relatively short-lived, and lasts only for about 6 months.

Passive Artificial Immunity: Here, antibodies are introduced to the body artificially after being obtained from another human or from an animal.

Immune serum or antiserum is obtained by actively immunizing an animal to the disease in question, and then removing the serum containing antibodies. This is refined and concentrated, and injected into patients as and when necessary.

Tetanus and diphtheria antitoxic sera or antitoxins are used to protect patients against these diseases. Antitoxins offer immediate but short-lived protection, usually not greater than three weeks. Therefore tetanus *antitoxin* is used for the immediate protection of patients who have already been exposed to the disease, for example those who have received serious and dirty wounds. However, tetanus *toxoid* is used to give long standing active immunity to those likely to be exposed to the tetanus bacillus some time in the future, for example building-site workers.

Combination Immunity

Nowadays combined preparations are administered to confer active immunity against several diseases at the same time, for example the triple injection against whooping cough, diphtheria, and tetanus.

Antibodies

Specific defence substances produced by the body in response to an attack by a specific substance, and carried in the blood. They will later help the body's defences only against that same substance. The cells associated with their formation are lymphocytes and plasma cells.

HYPERSENSITIVITY

A state in which the tissues respond in an abnormal way to the introduction of substances that normally cause little or no reaction in normal tissues. The two varieties of hypersensitivity are anaphylaxis and allergy.

Anaphylaxis

Hypersensitivity due to repeated injections of certain substances into the body. The first dose sensitizes the patient, and later injections produce an abnormal response.

Allergy

This results from exposure to pollens, dusts, and foods such as strawberries. Occasionally allergic responses follow the application of lipsticks and powders, and may even occur after the administration of penicillin.

QUESTIONS

1. Describe the various methods of sterilization used in dental practice.

2. How would you sterilize the following articles:—
a. A root-canal reamer ?
b. A dental handpiece ?
c. A gauze swab ?
d. An all-glass hypodermic syringe ?
e. A pair of extraction forceps ?

3. What are:—
a. Bacteria ?
b. Spores ?
c. Allergy ?
Discuss their importance in dental surgery.

4. Discuss the importance of the Hepatitis virus in dental surgery. How may its transmission be prevented?

CHAPTER VIII

THE DENTAL SURGERY ASSISTANT AND HER WORK

GONE are the days when the dental surgery assistant was just used for domestic chores and as appointment maker. Today she works intelligently as part of a team, and must understand the techniques required for the modern practice of dental surgery. This type of work therefore offers a much wider scope than ever before, and it is essential for the surgery assistant to adopt a scientific approach to her work. The actual duties vary according to the size and nature of the practice, but consist of some or all of the following:—

1. Arranging appointments and recalls.
2. Preparation and postoperative care of patients.
3. Preparation and sterilization of instruments and dressings.
4. Recording and charting of treatment on dictation by the dental surgeon.
5. Assisting the dentist in all dental operations, including local and general anaesthetics, fillings, impressions, and dental radiography.
6. Care of drugs used in the surgery.
7. Care and maintenance of surgery equipment.
8. Supervision of general cleanliness in all rooms used by patients.
9. Preparation and collection of private and National Health accounts. Keeping of books and patients' treatment records.
10. Attending to correspondence.
11. Preparation of wages and tax deductions.

The duties thus fall into three categories:—

1. Practice management.
2. Reception.
3. Chairside assistance.

PRACTICE MANAGEMENT

Good administration is very important, to make things easier for patients and dentist. Correspondence must be dealt with immediately. Letters, appointment sheets, records, recall cards, forms, and ledgers should be kept in a standardized filing system, to facilitate searches by other members of staff.

Some practices are run fully by the dental surgeon, but many delegate management to a dental surgery assistant, receptionist, or, in very large practices, to a practice manager or secretary. In any case the surgery assistant will play a large part.

The good administrator D.S.A. knows and understands all the work and tasks to be carried out in the surgery. She must have a sound knowledge of techniques and procedures, care and routine maintenance of equipment, ordering and keeping of stock, an understanding of the temperaments of all the surgery team and how to help them, and must be able to step in and fill any space when a member of the ancillary team is absent, except where a special professional skill is required.

RECEPTION OF PATIENTS

It is important to remember that the patient's first impression of a dental practice is formed by what is heard on the telephone, and later by what is seen of the premises and waiting room.

The Telephone

Answer promptly and efficiently, but with warmth and understanding. The caller may be nervous or in pain, and needs reassurance. A clear well-pronounced voice is essential. Give facts, not chat. 'Good morning, Mr. Brown's surgery. Can I help you?' Politeness and pleasantness cost nothing and bring rewards. Time is important to the caller and to you. Keep appointment book, note pad, and pencil by the telephone. Be prompt, to the point, and always polite. Never rely on your memory, no matter how good it is. Keep a written record of all calls. Do not disturb the dentist unnecessarily. If he has a patient in the chair he should not be disturbed without very good cause. Time is at a premium to the dentist in a busy general practice. Also he must study each patient individually and provide uninterrupted treatment if he is to maintain their goodwill. The dentist can always telephone back if the name, number, and message have been recorded. First names or initials are very important. As so many people have similar surnames, mistakes can easily be made.

A list of the most used numbers should be kept by the telephone and should include those likely to be required in an emergency, such as local doctors, ambulance stations, hospitals, and dental service engineer.

Booking of Appointments

A separate appointment book or list should be kept for each dentist in the practice. The length of appointments varies according to the

procedure and individual requirements of dentist and patient. Every
care must be exercised when making entries in the appointment book,
as it is around this that the whole practice revolves. Pencil is better
than pen so that mistakes and cancellations can easily be erased. Some
dentists send out 'notes' to their receptionist stating the length of time
required for the next visit or the procedure which is to be performed.
New patients should be informed which dentist is to be seen. Emphasize
the need for notifying the surgery at least 24 hours in advance if the
appointment cannot be kept.

The Receptionist

One of her biggest assets is an ever winning smile. An encouraging
and confident manner gives an impression of efficiency. The use of
people's names shows an interest in the individual. Very few patients
visit a dentist feeling full of confidence, so anything that can be done to
help them is invaluable. Human understanding is as important as any
technical skill. Courtesy, consideration, and attentive listening are
necessary *at all times*. The knowledge that one is doing an important
and worthwhile job helps to maintain high standards.

The Patient

What is said to patients within the first few minutes of arrival is
vital to the well-being and popularity of a practice. It can have a
lasting effect on their relationship with the practice and with dentistry
generally. Carefully avoid words such as 'drill' and 'pain'. Never
discuss treatment in the hearing of other patients. Tell the patient
your name and that of the dentist. This helps to establish a warm
relationship. Older patients and children may require special attention
and patience. One should show an interest in their problems, hobbies,
and families. Addressing them by name is preferable to terms such as
'dear' and 'sonny'.

Anxiety can be alleviated by a sympathetic approach. If patients
have wrong ideas about dentistry, do not belittle them. Give a firm
assurance that the dentist will understand their concern. It is unethical
to discuss members of staff with patients. Remember that other patients
may be able to overhear your conversation, and will get a very poor
impression both of you and of the practice. If a dentist falls behind with
appointments owing to unforeseen circumstances, explain this to waiting
patients.

When calling a patient into a surgery always introduce the dentist
and patient to each other. This commences a good relationship on both
sides and breaks down tension to some degree.

After treatment is finished see that the patient leaves the surgery feeling satisfied and comfortable. Do not keep them chatting unnecessarily. See that they have their next appointment and the surgery telephone number, in case they should need this.

The Waiting Room

A high standard of cleanliness is essential. Magazines should be kept up-to-date, and dog-eared reading matter should be discarded. Magazines should be tidily placed within sight and reach of all patients, young or old, tall or short. A low table is suitable for this purpose. Few extraneous articles should be in evidence. Posters, literature, and notices must be kept in a clean state, and should be renewed regularly.

A special children's corner makes young children feel wanted and important. Special paper on one wall, small chairs, jig-saw puzzles, books, and small toys all help to retain their interest while waiting.

IN THE SURGERY

Doors to surgery, waiting room, and recovery room must be kept closed. Drawers and cupboards in the surgery should be closed immediately after use. Tidiness is indicative of efficiency. Cupboards and drawers should be kept clean by lining with self-adhesive materials which can be wiped with a damp cloth. Linings should be renewed periodically.

Records, charts, radiographs, models, and photographs relating to the patient should be at hand. They should be given to the dentist before the patient enters the surgery. When the patient enters there should be no signs of instruments or materials used on the previous patient. The bracket table, cuspidor, head-rest, ends of spray bottles, air syringes and handpieces should be cleaned after each patient. Fresh and clean saliva ejectors and mouthwash beakers are essential. Patients often complain that everyone seems to use the same beaker. Thus, the disposable variety is appreciated. If the D.S.A. makes a good impression with these minor details the practice will get a good reputation for its standards. Observant patients watch out for quite ordinary details and can be very critical of what is seen.

Seat the patient in the chair, with back- and head-rests adjusted correctly. The back-rest top should be in line with the lower part of the shoulder-blades. The head-rest should aline with the base of the skull, so that the head is in line with the rest of the body. If the supine position is to be used, give the patient some idea of how the chair will be adjusted, so that no alarm is caused. If the dentist and assistant are to sit either side of the patient, this should be explained. Keep patients in mind throughout any preparation so that they know what is to take place and what is expected of them. Place a clean napkin around the patient's neck. Ensure that all instruments required for the operation are at hand, either on bracket table, trolley, or tray, as desired by the dentist. Be very aware of the dentist's routine with all his work so that his every need can be anticipated and met. He should not have to ask for equipment. A well-trained D.S.A. has everything in readiness. She must therefore be familiar with the operation to be performed, the instruments and materials to be used, and how to prepare them. She must remember that time and materials are costly.

In many busy practices one of the team is constantly at the chairside giving necessary assistance, while another assistant is responsible for materials, processing radiographs, and fetching and carrying instruments when required. Talking and noise of any kind is kept to a minimum during operative procedures.

The assistant who is acting as helper should constantly clear away used instruments and soiled materials, and should prepare the former for sterilization.

The use of dental materials is most important and these should be well understood and used correctly so that wastage does not occur. They are expensive to purchase. If the 'Directions for Use' are not adhered to, materials will often be wasted and, more important, the dentist's work will be ruined. It is good practice to keep a folder of all printed instructions so that they can be referred to when needed. The small amount of time spent in reading this literature saves much frustration, time, and money.

Dental suppliers are always prepared to advise on the use of materials and are naturally concerned when products do not appear to perform correctly. Their constant problem is that assistants become over-familiar with the materials and do not always follow the 'Directions for Use'. Therefore it is a sensible precaution when things go wrong to check that the correct procedure is being followed before complaining to the supplier.

Never adopt a slap happy attitude in the dental surgery. It is exacting work and precision is essential at all times.

FOUR-HANDED DENTISTRY

In four-handed dentistry the D.S.A. provides close support for the dentist, sitting on the opposite side of the patient. The actual position depends upon the operative procedure being performed, and upon the dentist's wishes. The surgery assistant places all new instruments firmly into the dentist's hands, ensuring that they are the correct way round for use. She takes away each instrument after it has been used. It is therefore important for the D.S.A. to have all instruments laid out in front of her, so that they are in reach. To ensure the speedy and efficient care of patients, the surgery assistant must be one step ahead of the dentist, so that the latter is not held up whilst, for example, the D.S.A. searches for a matrix holder. She must ensure that the correct rotating instrument is in the handpiece. The cavity is washed and aspirated to ensure that the site of operation is clean. Lips and cheeks are retracted so that the dentist can see what he is doing.

PERSONAL HYGIENE

Personal cleanliness is absolutely essential for all those coming into contact with patients. Spotless uniforms, clean and well-manicured nails, and hands which are smooth and clean are all essential. Cleanliness of the hands must never be neglected. Although the surgery assistant is always 'at the sink' the importance of a thorough washing technique cannot be too strongly emphasized. This should be done in full view of the patient. Washing helps to prevent the transfer of germs between patients, and ensures that bacteria picked up from a patient do not stay for too long in contact with your skin. If they do, and an instrument pricks the finger in this region, germs can pass into the body and cause an inflammatory lesion. Complete skin sterility is not possible, but running water and a bactericidal soap are fairly efficient. The nails should be scrubbed to remove any impacted amalgam as well as bacteria. After washing the hands they must be carefully dried. Application of a barrier hand cream helps to keep them smooth and supple. A good supply of soap, brushes, and clean towels is essential. Sinks must be kept spotlessly clean.

Hair should be carefully groomed, and jewellery should not be worn. Note that rings made of gold may be ruined by mercury. A good deodorant reduces unpleasant odours from perspiration which are encouraged by warm surgery conditions. Close contact with the public and other members of staff in confined areas calls for particular attention to body hygiene. Feet require very special care, especially in those suffering from excessive perspiration. Special powders and soaps can be used to reduce the problem. Stockings should be changed regularly to keep them dry. Shoes must allow air to circulate around the feet, give good support, and aid posture. Proper exercise and fresh air are essential for those working indoors. Walking, swimming, and dancing are excellent forms of exercise. 'Keep fit' classes are nowadays available at local educational institutions.

A well groomed and pleasant mannered assistant or receptionist is an invaluable asset to any surgery and its team of workers. She can influence others by her own manner and appearance.

MAINTENANCE OF SURGERY EQUIPMENT

The following schedule is recommended for maximum equipment efficiency. Reference should also be made to manufacturers' instruction booklets to ensure that all procedures are carried out in the correct way.

Daily

MORNING

Turn on mains water, electricity, gas, and air.
Switch on sterilizer.
Check oil level in reservoir of air turbine.
Move dental chair fully up and down.
Refill spray bottles as necessary.

NIGHT

Clean aspirator and saliva ejector systems with a proprietary cleaner.
Empty cuspidor trap (*not* down cuspidor arm).
Clean and lubricate straight and right-angle handpieces.
Lubricate air turbine handpieces in accordance with the manufacturers' instructions.

(It is strongly recommended that the foregoing items should receive attention as soon as the last patient has gone, rather than leaving them all night.)

Turn off compressor and sterilizer.
Extinguish any flames.
Finally, release water pressure on flexible tubings and ensure that water, electricity, gas, and air are turned off before leaving the surgery, both at night and during lunch periods.

Weekly

Clean enamel and plating using polish recommended by the manufacturers.
Lubricate moving parts of equipment with *one or two* drops of oil, or a smear of grease as appropriate.
Blow moisture out of turbine air lines in accordance with manufacturers' instructions.
Flush out spray-bottle nozzles with clear water.
Pour two or three pints of warm soda water or special proprietary cleaner down cuspidor (with waste trap removed) to clean waste system.

Monthly

Drain compressor tank of water accumulation by means of draincock at base of tank; change air filters and renew pads when necessary, drain moisture extractor of turbine outfit (if in doubt consult manufacturers' instructions).

Lubricate compressor pump mechanism, if necessary.

Lubricate all motor bearings *sparingly*, unless of self-oiling type.

Check and clean commutator. Check carbon brushes for wear.

Change oil and clean control box of turbine in accordance with manufacturer's instructions.

Recommended List of Spares to be carried

Carbon brushes, turbine oil and cleaners, compressor oil, turbine chucks, enamel and plating polish, set of fuses, pilot bulbs, operating-light bulbs, engine cords, or other items as indicated in the manufacturers' instructions.

Instrument Care

Dental handpieces must be regularly maintained. Standard ones should be frequently oiled. It is useful to run them in oiling and cleaning fluids. If they get wet in use handpieces should be dismantled and dried. Worn bearings should be renewed when necessary, and chucks on straight handpieces should be adjusted. Air turbine handpieces should receive oil from a reservoir. The oil level should be checked to ensure that it is correct, after which one should ensure that an oil mist is reaching the bearings of the handpiece. The best method is to hold the bur still whilst allowing air to blow oil through the system. Plastic chucks should be renewed when necessary.

Sharpen chisels and excavators on an oiled Arkansas stone, or arrange for them to be resharpened by a dental supply house (*Fig.* 34).

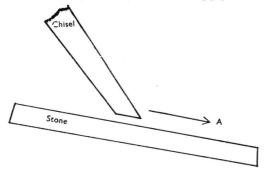

Fig. 34.—Sharpening an enamel chisel by pushing it along the stone towards A.

Meticulously cleanse and sterilize burs and hand instruments. Amalgam carriers should be thoroughly cleared while the amalgam is soft. Should the residue become hard, metal nozzles may be cleared by heating gently. Surplus amalgam should be kept under water in containers, to prevent mercury vapour intoxication. It can be sold later as scrap metal.

If the dental surgery assistant has any doubt regarding these tasks, she should ask the dentist to give her a demonstration of the correct techniques.

REQUISITION OF SUPPLIES

It is essential to order sensibly so as to take advantage of suppliers' quantity rates. Do not order large quantities of items which are seldom used, especially if they have a limited shelf life. Establish a simple basic stock-and-order system to ensure against running out of essential supplies. Maintain a current 'want list' of surgery items, and add items immediately stocks get low.

Use the approved practice system for ordering stores, and ensure that a record is kept of all items ordered. Full use should be made of manufacturers' catalogues to ensure that the correct descriptions are used. This identification speeds delivery. When goods received have been checked, delivery notes should be initialled and the original order ticked off. Payment is usually made on a monthly basis to gain maximum trading discounts.

Stock cupboards should not be overloaded and must be kept clean and tidy. Bottles must be neatly and clearly labelled, with particular attention being paid to any containing poisonous or corrosive substances. Antidotes for such medicaments must be at hand. Contents of any unlabelled bottles should be thrown away to avoid an accident.

CONSENT FOR TREATMENT

Any treatment, as opposed to examination, may be classed as an assault unless the patient has given permission for this treatment, preferably in writing. Parents should sign for children under the age of sixteen years. A special written consent should be obtained prior to the administration of a general anaesthetic.

QUESTIONS

1. Summarize briefly what you consider to be the duties of a surgery assistant other than those of assisting the operator. Explain the importance of these duties.

2. What is your normal procedure in answering a telephone call at

your practice ? How would you deal with:—
    a. A new patient ?
    b. A patient wishing to make an appointment for extraction under general anaesthesia ?
    c. A patient who wishes to cancel an appointment ?
    d. A patient who has failed to keep an appointment ?
    3. Discuss the part the dental chairside assistant may play in the building up of a successful and efficient dental practice.
    4. Give an account of the role of a D.S.A. in four-handed dentistry.

CHAPTER IX

RECORDS AND CHARTING

IT is essential for the dentist to have accurate records relating to the present state of patients' mouths, past treatment completed, and treatment still required. A knowledge of past treatment is often useful in planning the present course of treatment. Also, records are increasingly being used to aid identification of crash and murder victims, so one must be meticulous in the keeping of such records.

CHARTING

Charting is a shorthand method of recording dental conditions on paper, so that it can be understood at a later date both by the same dentist and by others. One must therefore be able to indicate the presence or absence of individual teeth, whether they have caries or fillings, and whether any need to be extracted.

RIGHT
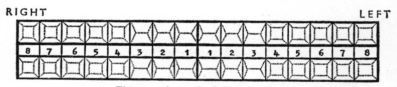
LEFT

Fig. 35.—A standard dental chart.

Fig. 35 shows an example of a standard type of dental chart. One immediately notices that right and left are reversed. This is because the chart is really a map of the patient's mouth as viewed from in front. The patient's left at this time is on the dentist's right. The numbers 1 to 8 indicate which permanent tooth is referred to when charting, starting from the central incisor and working back to the wisdom teeth. The upper boxes refer to the maxillary teeth and the lower ones to the mandibular teeth. That segment of each box closest to the numbers indicates the lingual surfaces—the upper part of mandibular boxes, the lower part of maxillary ones. The part furthest from the numbers indicates buccal surfaces. When referring to deciduous teeth the numbers are replaced by the letters A, B, C, D, and E.

Premolars and Molars

Posterior teeth have five surfaces. *Fig.* 36 illustrates a diagram of an upper right tooth. In lower teeth buccal and lingual are interchanged. A left tooth would have mesial and distal reversed. The signs for cavities and fillings can be indicated on any surface.

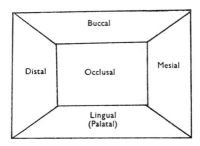

Fig. 36.—Diagram of an upper right molar or premolar tooth.

Incisors and Canines

Anterior teeth have four surfaces plus an incisal tip. These are indicated diagrammatically in *Fig.* 37.

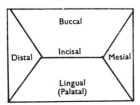

Fig. 37.—Diagram of an upper right incisor or canine.

Charting Signs

Fig. 38 shows the common signs used as abbreviations on dental charts.

O	Caries	⫲	Tooth fractured
●	Filling		Direction of movement of teeth
⊙	Unsound restoration (needs to be refilled)	AR	Artificial tooth present
—	Tooth missing at examination	CR	Crown present
/	Tooth to be extracted	BR	Bridge retainer present
×	Tooth has been extracted	BP	Bridge pontic present
+	Root present	RF	Tooth root filled
U	Tooth unerupted		

Fig. 38.—Some commonly used charting signs.

Written Signs

These are used in the treatment notes section of a dental record rather than in the charting part.

$\llcorner$ upper left (remember this as L for left)

e.g., $\underline{4}$ = upper left first premolar

$\lrcorner$ upper right

e.g. $\mathrm{A}\underline{|}$ = upper right first deciduous incisor

$\ulcorner$ lower left

e.g., $\overline{|8}$ = lower left third molar

$\urcorner$ lower right

e.g., $\overline{\mathrm{C}|}$ = lower right deciduous canine

Examples of written signs in use are:—

$\overline{|6_0}$ = occlusal cavity in lower left first molar;

$\dfrac{^{m}1|}{|5_b}$ = mesial cavity in upper right central, buccal cavity in lower left second premolar;

$\underline{6|}$ A.R. = upper right first molar filled with an amalgam restoration.

FORMAT OF A DENTAL RECORD

In addition to charting teeth, dentists will usually put the following sections on a patient's record card, often in a very abbreviated form:—

1. *Names* (first and surname).

2. *Address.*

3. *Telephone numbers* (home and work).

4. *Complains of* (*symptoms*).
   Why has the patient come? pain, bleeding gums, bad breath or taste, swelling?

5. *History of present complaint.*
   How long has the patient had the present symptoms, has he had them before, what makes them worse or better?

6. *Past dental history.*
   What sort of treatment has the patient had previously? Does he bleed excessively when a tooth is removed? Has he had a local or general anaesthetic?

7. *General medical history.*
   Is the patient under the care of his doctor or of a hospital? Is he receiving any drug therapy? Does he suffer from lesions of the heart and circulation, or respiratory system?

8. *On examination.*
    What the dentist sees (signs):—
    a. Patient's general appearance.
    b. The face, head, and neck.
    c. Intra-oral (within the mouth).
9. *Aids to diagnosis.*
    Study models, radiographs, and photographs.
10. *Diagnosis.*
    What exactly is wrong with the patient ?
11. *Treatment plan.*
    What should be done to complete treatment to the best advantage
    of the patient ?
    e.g., a. Scale and polish.
         b. Root canal therapy |2.
         c. Conservation $\dfrac{65\,|\,3}{1\,|\,6}$.
         d. Bridge 4|.
         e. Partial lower denture.

QUESTIONS

1   a. What are the disadvantages of failing to keep accurate dental
records ?
    b. What means are used to detect carious cavities in teeth ?
Describe a method of charting and recording these cavities.
    2. What is dental shorthand for:—
    a. Upper left permanent central incisor ?
    b. Lower right deciduous canine ?
    c. Upper right first premolar for extraction ?
    d. Lower left wisdom tooth unerupted ?
    3. Discuss the information recorded on a typical dental record card.
    4. In what ways can a dentist assist the police in identifying a dead
body?

CHAPTER X

FUNCTIONS AND IDENTIFICATION OF INSTRUMENTS

It is absolutely essential for chairside assistants to know the names of all instruments to be found in the dental surgery. When the dentist asks for an instrument he does not expect to have to show her what is required.

Although most instruments have a number, the name is much more important, except when working with the occasional dentist who only asks for them by the number. This is often stamped on the instrument, so there is less difficulty involved in identification. Another method of identification is to put different coloured sleeves on different types of instruments.

In this chapter we outline the uses of instruments and illustrate some of the commoner ones. Manufacturers' catalogue pictures should be kept by you when learning the names. The only way to memorize them is to handle the instruments, perhaps getting a dentist or another surgery assistant to question you on names and functions.

FUNCTION OF INSTRUMENTS

Abrasive cones, disks, wheels (green): Crown and inlay preparations, grinding teeth.

Abrasive cones, disks, wheels (white): Used with petroleum jelly to polish silicate fillings.

Amalgam carrier, straight (Hampel): Transfer of amalgam to cavities.

Amalgam carrier, right-angle (R.A.): Transfer of amalgam to less accessible cavities.

Atomizer: Bottle for spraying water, disinfectants, etc., on to oral tissues.

Burs: Removal of decay and surrounding tooth structure.

Burs, finishing: To smooth the junction between enamel and filling, ensuring that no rough edges remain to hold food particles against the tooth.

Broaches, barbed: Removal of pulp contents from root canals.

Broaches, smooth: Detection of shape and length of root canals.

Carvers: Shaping of amalgam fillings and wax patterns to conform to the tooth outline.

Chisels, Coupland: Expansion of socket and breakdown of periodontal membrane prior to extraction.

Chisels, enamel: Removal of unsupported enamel prisms during cavity preparation. Similarly hatchets and hoes. Gingival margin trimmers have a similar function in the gingival region of proximal boxes.

Excavators: Removal of carious dentine.

Elevators: Removal of roots and teeth by rotating the point against root.

Elevators, periosteal: Reflection of flaps during apicectomy and subperiosteal curettage.

Files, bone: Contouring bone during alveolectomy and surgical operations.

Forceps: Extraction of teeth.

Forceps, pocket-marking: Indicating amount of tissue to be removed during gingivectomy.

Forceps, rongeur: Removal of alveolar bone following extractions and during alveolotomy.

Gags: To open the mouth of anaesthetized patients, and to enable the operator to change to the opposite side.

Handpieces: Hold rotating burs and mandrels during dental operations:—

    a. Straight; for anterior teeth.

    b. Contra angle; general purpose.

Knives, gingivectomy: Removal of hyperplastic gingival tissue.

Lancet: Incision of abscess.

Mandrels: Means of holding unmounted stones, discs, and wheels in a handpiece.

Matrix bands: Allow amalgam to be packed into cavities that are open on one side. It would otherwise fall out.

Plastics (flat and round): Insertion of cements and silicate fillings.

Pluggers: Compression of amalgam into cavities, forcing out excess mercury.

Probes: Detection of caries and rough edges on fillings and inlays.

Probes, Briault: Detection of interproximal decay.

Probes, Moon's: Detection of loose bone and roots in sockets.

Probes, pocket-measuring: To detect depth of pocket around periodontally involved teeth.

Props: Hold mouth open during extractions under general anaesthesia.

Reamers: Enlarge the inside of root canals until only healthy dentine remains (files are then used to smooth the walls).

Rotary paste fillers: Spin root filling and dressing materials towards the canal apex.

Rubber dam: Prevents entry of moisture to a cavity, especially prior to insertion of silicate fillings, and during root-canal therapy.

Rubber dam clamps: Hold dam on teeth.

Rubber dam forceps: Aid placement of clamps on teeth.

Rubber dam frame: Holds dam in position around mouth.

Saliva ejector: Removes saliva and water from mouth; otherwise the patient would have to be continually swallowing or choking.

Scaler: Removal of calculus.

Scissors, crown and collar: Shaping copper rings and stainless-steel crowns.

Spatulas, agate: Mixing silicate cements.

Spatulas, chrome-cobalt: Multipurpose mixing.

Spatulas, metal: Mixing oxyphosphate and similar cements.

Syringe: Means of introducing local anaesthetic into the tissues.

Syringe, chip: Blows debris and moisture from cavities prior to filling them.

Syringe, water: For washing out extraction sockets.

Trays: Hold impression materials.

Tweezers, college: Holding dressings, cotton-wool, etc.

ILLUSTRATIONS OF INSTRUMENTS

1. Instruments required for Detection and Treatment of Caries

a. PROBES

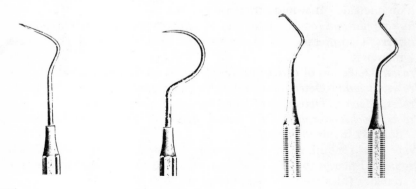

Straight (routine use)   Sickle (for anterior teeth)   Both ends of Briault probe No. 11
(for interproximal decay)

b. CHISELS, ETC.

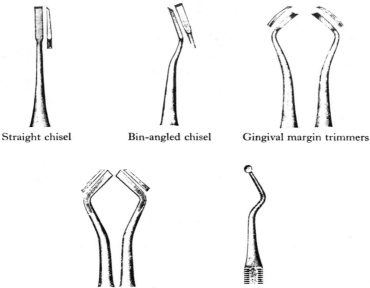

Straight chisel   Bin-angled chisel   Gingival margin trimmers

Enamel hatchets   Excavator

c. BURS

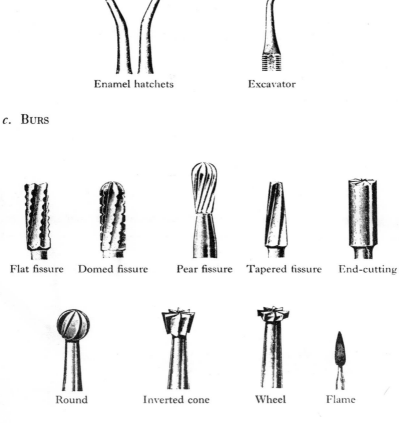

Flat fissure   Domed fissure   Pear fissure   Tapered fissure   End-cutting

Round   Inverted cone   Wheel   Flame

2. Insertion of Amalgam Fillings

a. MATRIX BANDS AND HOLDERS

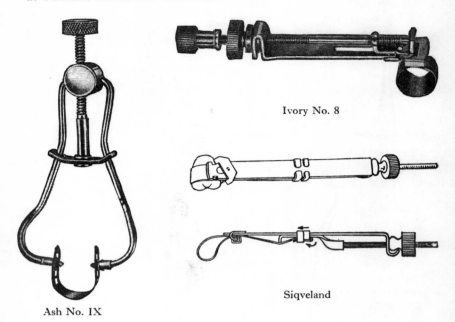

Ivory No. 8

Siqveland

Ash No. IX

b. AMALGAM CARRIERS

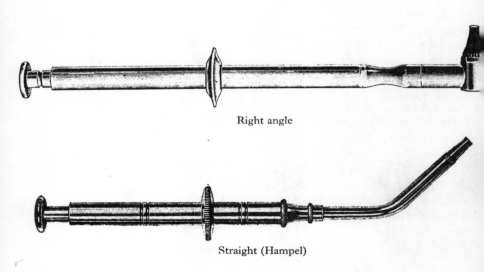

Right angle

Straight (Hampel)

3. Amalgam Instruments

Double-ended flat plastic and flat plugger

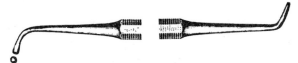

Round and pointed plastics

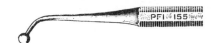

Burnisher

4. Amalgam Carvers

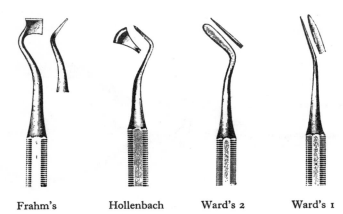

Frahm's   Hollenbach   Ward's 2   Ward's 1

5. Isolation of Teeth from Saliva

a. RUBBER DAM FRAME

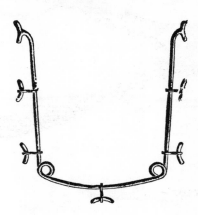

b. CLAMPS

Molar

Premolar

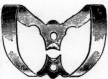

Incisor

c. CLAMP HOLDER

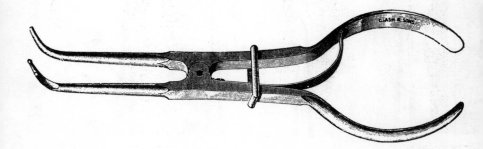

d. RUBBER DAM PUNCH

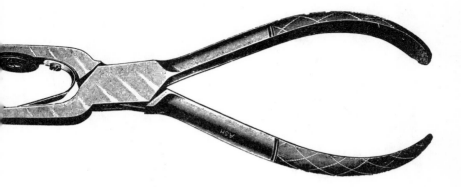

6. Extraction Forceps

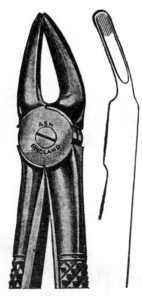

Upper Read's (canines,
premolars, roots)

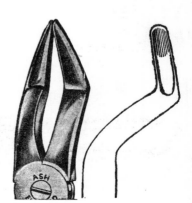

Upper bayonets (awkwardly
placed wisdom teeth)

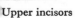

Upper incisors

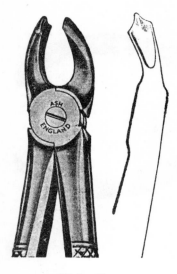

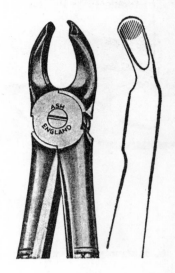

Right side   Left side

Upper molars

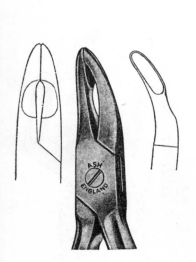

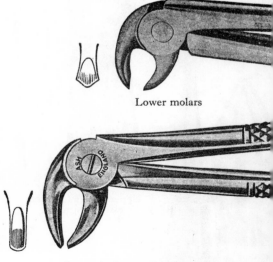

Lower molars

Rongeur's No. 4   Lower incisors, premolars, roots

7. Root Elevators

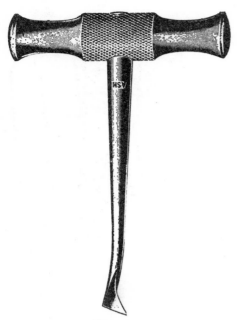

Winter's

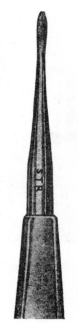

Straight Warwick James

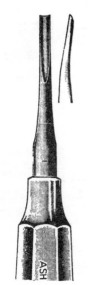

upland's osseous chisel

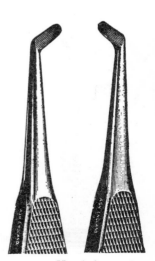

Hospital

8. Mouth Prop and Gag

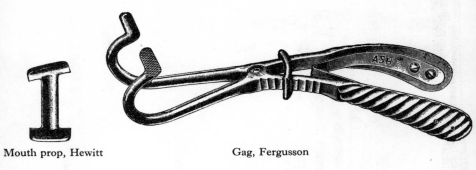

Mouth prop, Hewitt   Gag, Fergusson

9. Scalers

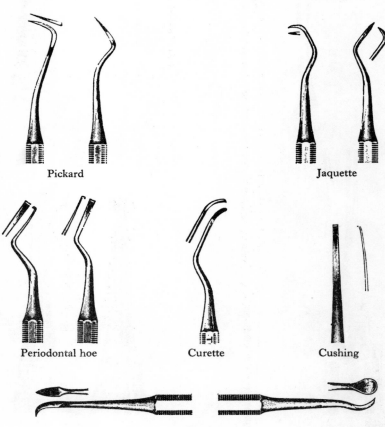

Pickard   Jaquette

Periodontal hoe   Curette   Cushing

Cumine

10. Gingivectomy Instruments

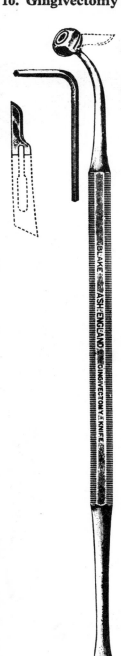

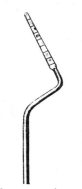

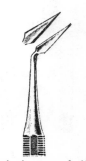

Pocket-measuring probe   Fish gingivectomy knife

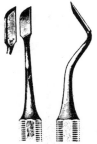

Fox gingivectomy knife

Periosteal elevator   Blake's universal knife

11. Instruments for Handpieces

a. MANDRELS

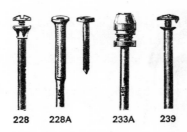

228   228A   233A   239

b. UNMOUNTED GREEN ABRASIVE STONES

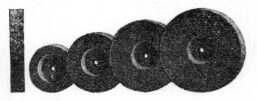

c. UNMOUNTED GREEN ABRASIVE DISKS

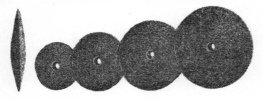

d. MOUNTED GREEN ABRASIVE STONES, DISKS, AND POINTS

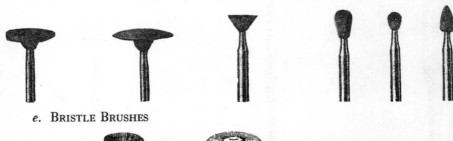

e. BRISTLE BRUSHES

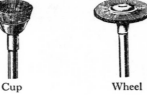

Cup   Wheel   Tooth-polishing

QUESTIONS

1. What instruments and other items of apparatus would you lay out for:—

   a. The removal of a buried root ?

   b. The insertion of a silicate filling with isolation of the tooth by rubber dam ?

2. Describe the various types of instruments which are used in dental handpieces. Give the uses of those you mention and briefly comment on their care and sterilization.

3. How would you clean and oil a contra-angled handpiece ?

4. Write notes on each of the following, indicating the circumstances in which they are used:—

   a. Periosteal elevator.

   b. Chrome cobalt spatula.

   c. Copper band.

   d. Rotary root canal filler.

CHAPTER XI

PROPERTIES AND USES OF DENTAL MATERIALS

IT is only with a full knowledge of the properties of materials that one can use them to the best advantage. When mixing dental materials due regard should be paid to the instructions supplied by manufacturers, as it is only in this way that the correct properties will be attained. All manufacturers want the best results to be obtained from their products so that dentists will continue to purchase them in the future.

IDEAL RESTORATIVE MATERIALS

They should:—

1. Be non-toxic and non-injurious to the dental and oral tissues.
2. Be strong and hard, but not brittle.
3. Not dissolve in the oral fluids.
4. Be easy to manipulate, and be adaptable to the tooth.
5. Match the colour of the tooth.
6. Expand and contract to the same degree as do tooth tissues with heat and cold.
7. Not expand or contract on setting.
8. Not set too rapidly, in order to allow sufficient time for manipulation.
9. Set fairly rapidly after insertion into the cavity.
10. Set in the presence of slight quantities of saliva.
11. Not change in form after placement in the teeth.
12. Make it possible to finish the restoration flush with the tooth surface.
13. Take and maintain a high degree of polish.
14. Be tasteless and odourless.
15. Not conduct heat or cold to the dentine and pulp.

The main restorative materials used are amalgam, silicate, acrylic, porcelain, gold, and stainless steel.

AMALGAM

Uses

1. Posterior fillings where aesthetics are of less importance.
2. Anterior fillings in mouths highly susceptible to caries, where other materials are rapidly attacked.

PROPERTIES

Amalgam alloy and mercury are mixed (amalgamated) prior to use. Alloy is a mixture of:—

Silver	68 per cent
Tin	26 per cent
Copper	5 per cent
Zinc	1 per cent

The function of each is:—

Silver: strength, colour, correct expansion.
Tin: ease of manipulation, increased flow, slower setting time.
Copper: hardness, increased setting time.
Zinc: increased dimensional stability, ease of working.

It is essential to use the correct proportions of alloy and mercury in accordance with the manufacturer's instructions otherwise incorrect properties will be obtained. Excess mercury causes weak amalgam with excessive expansion. Insufficient mercury causes brittle amalgam, rapid setting, lack of plasticity, and excessive contraction. It is therefore difficult to handle and pack into a cavity.

TECHNIQUES OF AMALGAMATION

1. Trituration of alloy and mercury with a pestle and mortar until the silvery mass clings to the side of the glass mortar. The pestle should be held in a 'pen-grip'.

2. By kneading them in a thick rubber finger-stall.

3. By vibrating them in an automatic amalgamator, for which purpose the constituents may be obtained pre-dispensed in capsules.

At least one death has been reported from excessive mercury intoxication, and fumes from mercury droplets left continuously on floors and bracket tables have been condemned as a source of danger to those working in surgeries. Waste amalgam and squeezed-out mercury should be kept under water to stop vapour getting into the atmosphere. Under no circumstances should the material be allowed to contact the skin. It has been known for operators to contract dermatitis. Moisture from the skin, e.g., with mulling in the hand, or from saliva leads to expansion of amalgam. This in turn causes pain, due to pressure on dentine overlying the pulp. Expansion out of the cavity leads to the formation of food-retaining edges, resulting in secondary or recurrent caries. Water also causes lower strength.

After mixing, the amalgam is sometimes mulled in a finger-stall. Excess mercury is then removed by squeezing the mix in a gauze napkin, held between the fingers and thumb. The mercury is dropped into water contained in a bottle. Unused or waste amalgam is also placed in this bottle. This waste material can be sold when sufficient has accumulated.

Over-trituration:
1. Faster set.
2. High expansion.
3. Weakness.

As amalgam is a metal that conducts heat and cold, a lining is often placed between the underlying sensitive dentine and the filling.

AESTHETIC RESTORATIVE MATERIALS

Three major types of material have been developed for use as aesthetic anterior filling materials:—
1. Silicates.
2. Acrylic resins.
3. Composites.

SILICATES (SYNTHETICS)

USES

1. Semi-permanent restorations in the front of the mouth as the colour and translucency match the natural tooth substance.
2. Facing gold crowns at the chairside.

PROPERTIES

Silicates consist of a liquid and a powder.

Powder is composed of silica, alumina, flux, lime, zinc oxide.

Liquid is phosphoric acid, water, aluminium, and zinc phosphates. The liquid rapidly takes up or gives off water according to the humidity (water content of the atmosphere). It is important that bottles should be kept tightly stoppered when not in use, as changes in water content affect the setting reaction. Unfortunately, silicates are not long lasting. Some are supplied in pre-dispensed capsules. In this case the liquid is contained in a membrane, which is ruptured just before use, by squeezing in a special press. This brings liquid and powder into contact, after which they are mixed in a mechanical mixer for about 10 seconds.

TECHNIQUE

1. A thick glass slab is cooled with cold water and dried. Thick glass retains the coolness for a long period of time, allowing a longer mixing time.

2. The required quantities of liquid and powder are placed on the slab. It is important to hold the dropper vertically to ensure that the correct amount of liquid is dispensed.

3. The powder is divided into four sections, each approximately half the size of the next section.

4. The largest pile of powder is speedily mixed into the liquid followed by rapid addition of the other three sections until a dough-like consistency is obtained. A maximum quantity of powder added in this way gives maximum strength and adaptability. As soon as setting begins, manipulation must be stopped.

An agate, chrome-cobalt, or bone spatula may be used. Ordinary metal ones are affected by the acidic liquid. A special glass slab is kept for silicates. Remnants of other materials could contaminate and interfere with the durability of silicate fillings.

As silicates are affected by moisture, a rubber dam is often placed on the tooth before inserting the filling.

Silicate mixtures are acidic and would affect the pulp if no lining were used. As they rapidly dry out and take up stains during setting, a coating of special varnish is usually applied to newly-inserted fillings.

ACRYLIC RESINS

USES OF HEAT-CURED RESINS

1. Denture base materials and artificial teeth.
2. Removable orthodontic appliances.
3. Crowns.

USES OF COLD-CURED (AUTOGENOUS) RESINS

1. Fillings in anterior teeth (tend to shrink and discolour).
2. Repairing dentures and orthodontic appliances.
3. Special trays.

Acrylics consist basically of a powder and a liquid. In addition the cold-cure variety also has a catalyst.

Powder: Methyl methacrylate polymer.

Liquid: Monomer.

Catalyst: Cream or liquid chemical accelerator. This speeds up the setting process for cold-cure acrylic, as does heat for the other variety of resin.

TECHNIQUE

Measured quantities of catalyst and liquid monomer are rapidly mixed with a glass spatula in a glass or porcelain container. Powder is added until it forms a layer on top, and all the ingredients are then mixed to form a dough-like consistency. As the mixture is affected by moisture, fillings are often placed in teeth under rubber dam protection.

COMPOSITE RESTORATIVE MATERIALS

These are combinations of two or more materials combined either to improve the properties of one constituent, or to yield a material with properties different to those from which it is made.

Most composites have a polymer system called Bis-GMA, based upon the organic compound Bisphenol A Glycidyl Methacrylate.

USES

Restorations where aesthetics is of prime importance.

PROPERTIES

Composites are supplied in four basic forms:—
Two pastes.
Paste and liquid.
Powder and liquid.
Paste and powder.

Paste–Paste System

One paste is the universal or base paste, the other is the catalyst. Some manufacturers supply tints to adjust the shade.

Base contains Bis-GMA, treated inorganic particles, pigments, and accelerator.

Catalyst also contains Bis-GMA and inorganic particles, plus a catalyst.

TECHNIQUE

One end of a disposable plastic or wooden spatula is used to stir the universal paste. The other end is used for the catalyst, in order to prevent contamination and therefore hardening in the container. Equal amounts of each are placed on a pad and they are mixed for about 30 seconds, depending upon the maker's instructions. An agate, wooden or plastic spatula may be used, but *never* a metal one. Small amounts of the metal may contaminate and discolour the composite. Tint can be added to the universal paste to adjust the colour prior to adding catalyst. Only when the latter is added will hardening begin.

After about a further minute the material starts to harden, and no more manipulation can take place either outside or within the mouth.

Paste–Liquid System

Paste contains Bis-GMA, treated inorganic particles, pigments and catalyst.

Liquid is an organic one containing the accelerator.

TECHNIQUE

The required amount of paste is placed on a mixing pad and a depression is made in the centre. Liquid catalyst is dropped into the depression, and then mixed by folding it into the paste with an agate spatula, for about 30 seconds.

Care must be taken to avoid prolonged contact of liquid or mixed paste with the skin.

Another product, initiated by ultra-violet light, is also available. In this case the paste contains dimethacrylate, catalyst, pigments, and inorganic particles. A drop of initiator is added to the paste and the two are mixed. If protected from light the mixture should remain workable for three months. Hardening takes place by exposure to the UV light.

Powder–Liquid System

Powder may be treated inorganic particles alone, or may contain as much as 75 per cent methylmethacrylate polymer. It also contains a catalyst and pigments.

Liquid may be Bis-GMA diluted with methacrylate monomers to reduce the viscosity, or it may be another dimethacrylate. The liquid also contains an accelerator.

TECHNIQUE

The powder and liquid are supplied in bottles and pre-dispensed capsules. Various shades are available. Powder and liquid are dispensed with a small plastic scoop and a dropper bottle, and then mixed with a spatula for 15 seconds.

Paste–Powder System

Paste contains dimethacrylate plus inorganic particles, pigments, and catalysts.

Powder consists of micro-capsules of the accelerator deposited on the surface of the *mixing pad* itself.

TECHNIQUE

The paste is pressed hard on the pad in order to break the microscopic capsules. Mixing is for 15 seconds.

PORCELAIN

Uses

1. Artificial teeth.
2. Crowns.
3. Occasionally inlays.

Porcelain provides a better colour match than acrylic. It is harder and therefore does not wear down so rapidly. However, it does tend to be brittle, and is liable to shatter if subjected to a sudden and excessive force. It cannot be prepared at the chairside because it must be cooked in a high temperature oven.

GOLD

Used as foil or cast metal. Both take and retain a high polish.

Foil

Thin pieces of pure gold are placed into the cavity, one on top of another. Each is joined to its partner by cohesion, using very firm pressure (known as cold welding). This technique for small fillings is seldom used now.

Cast Gold

Three types of gold alloy are used for casting; hard, medium, and soft according to the function required. Hardness depends upon the different metals added to the basic gold during manufacture. Cast gold is used for inlays, crowns, posts, denture bases, bridges, and clasps.

The Ideal Inlay or Crown Alloy

1. High corrosion resistance (i.e., not liable to attack by oral fluids, food, medicines, etc.), as it cannot often be taken out for cleaning.
2. Slightly soft, to allow some adaptation (burnishing) of gold at the margins, to cover over the thin layer of cement between inlay and tooth.

Soft Inlays

For restorations which are well supported by tooth structure, and which do not have to resist large biting forces, e.g., Class V inlays. The edges are easily burnished.

Medium Inlays

These are stronger and harder. They allow very slight burnishing, usually a few days after insertion when the surface layer of cement at the edges has washed away. They are used far more than soft gold inlays.

Hard Inlays

These give great strength and are very valuable for thin sections, e.g., basket crowns and abutments for fixed bridges. As no burnishing is possible extreme accuracy is needed.

STAINLESS STEEL

Occasionally used for crowns on very badly broken down deciduous teeth, and as a temporary protective cover on fractured anterior teeth. It is also used for denture bases, orthodontic bands, clasps, and springs.

DENTAL CEMENTS

Uses
1. Temporary or semi-permanent fillings.
2. To cement in position crowns, inlays, and bridges.
3. To line cavities in order to prevent thermal or chemical damage to the pulp.
4. Support of remaining weak tooth structure.
The main cements used are:—
1. Zinc oxide and eugenol.
2. Accelerated zinc oxide–eugenol.
3. Special zinc oxide–eugenol products.
4. EBA cements.
5. Zinc polycarboxylates.
6. Zinc and copper phosphates.
7. Glass–ionomer (ASPA) cements.

Zinc Oxide and Eugenol

Uses
1. Protective cavity sub-linings (over which an oxyphosphate lining is placed for resistance to packing and biting pressure).
2. Sedative or obtundent (soothing) dressings (eugenol relieves painful hyperaemia of the pulp).
3. Temporary fillings.
4. Pulp caps.
5. Root canal fillings.
6. Periodontal packs.

Properties
1. Consists of a liquid and powder:—

Powder consists of zinc oxide, magnesium oxide, and zinc acetate (an accelerator).
Liquid contains eugenol, olive oil, and acetic acid as an accelerator.
2. Sedative action on pulp.
3. Prevents conduction of heat to pulp.
4. Very soluble in water.
5. Very weak.
6. Bacteriostatic.

TECHNIQUE

Four parts of powder are mixed with 1 of liquid until a putty-like consistency is obtained. This sets slowly in the presence of moisture, including saliva. If kept reasonably dry in a container (with a dehydrating agent such as calcium chloride), it will remain ready for use throughout the day. This saves mixing some each time it is required.

Accelerated Zinc Oxide–Eugenol

Quick-setting mixtures contain a resin to speed up the setting time from the normal twelve hours to five minutes. They are prepared and used in the same way as normal zinc oxide mixtures. However, they are not displaced if amalgam is condensed directly on to it, so no other lining needs to be placed between the two materials.

Special Zinc Oxide–Eugenol Products

Some contain antibiotics such as tetracyclines, plus steroids. They are used for root canal therapy and pulp capping.

EBA Cements

PROPERTIES

EBA (ortho-ethoxybenzoic acid) consists of a powder and liquid:—
Powder contains zinc oxide, fused quartz and hydrogenated rosin.
Liquid consists of eugenol and O-ethoxybenzoic acid.
This material shows considerably increased mechanical properties over normal zinc oxide–eugenol cements.

TECHNIQUE

As much as seven parts of powder are added to one of liquid in order to improve the mechanical properties.

Zinc Polycarboxylates

USES
1. Cementation of fixed orthodontic appliances.
2. Cavity linings.

PROPERTIES

1. They originally consisted of:—
   a. Powdered zinc oxide with small quantities of magnesium oxide.
   b. Liquid of approximately 40 per cent aqueous solution of poly-acrylic acid.
   Recent materials have included:—
   a. Products with two liquids of different viscosities; a thinner liquid for cementing and a viscous one for cavity lining.
   b. Two products with polyacrylic acid in the powder. The liquids for these contain 95 per cent water. One product is encapsulated for mechanical mixing.
   c. Encapsulated material with about 43 per cent alumina in the powder.
   d. One product with a polymer slightly different to polyacrylic acid.
   e. One cement contains stannous fluoride.
2. Very adhesive to clean dry enamel.
3. Saliva considerably reduces the adhesive strength.
4. Adheres better to a smooth surface than to a rough one (in contrast to zinc phosphates).
5. Adhesion to dentine is not as good as to enamel.
6. Does not adhere well to gold or porcelain.
7. Adheres to stainless steel.
8. Little irritant effect on the pulp.
9. More soluble than zinc phosphate materials.
10. Good thermal insulation properties.

TECHNIQUE

The liquid and powder must be thoroughly mixed as quickly as possible, as the cement will not stick to tooth substance once setting has begun. This can be a little difficult as the liquid is somewhat thicker than in most cements. Once ' cobwebbing ' occurs the mix must not be used.

Zinc Oxyphosphate

USES

1. Cavity lining.
2. Cementing crowns, bridges, and inlays.

PROPERTIES

1. Consists of a powder and a liquid:—
   Powder is mainly zinc oxide, plus magnesium oxide, and other oxides.

Liquid is mostly an aqueous solution of phosphoric acid.

2. Highly acidic, so deep cavities require a sub-lining to protect the pulp.

3. Stronger than zinc oxide–eugenol.

4. Good thermal insulator.

5. Does not adhere well to enamel or dentine.

TECHNIQUE

The required amount of liquid and powder are mixed with a stainless-steel spatula on a clean, cool glass slab. The quantity of powder incorporated varies according to the purpose for which it is required:—

a. As a lining, thick mix for strength and lessened risk of pulpal damage as there is a lower proportion of acid.

b. As a cement, slightly thinner to provide a reduced thickness of cement between crown and tooth.

Powder is added slowly, using a little at a time from three or four heaps, to slow the setting rate. Each heap is mixed in thoroughly before the next is added. The spatula is rapidly moved in circles around the slab ensuring that no unmixed particles of powder are left. Spatulation must cease by the time setting begins or the mix will be weakened. One minute is the usual time for spatulation.

As with all materials, the correct quantities of liquid and powder should have been placed on the slab. This assessment of amounts gets easier with practice. Under no circumstances should any be returned to the bottle as it will be contaminated, and so will affect subsequent mixes.

After use the slab should be placed in warm water to facilitate cleaning. The glass should not be scratched or later mixes of cement will tend to stick to it.

Stoppers must be replaced immediately on bottles, as water is lost or absorbed according to atmospheric humidity. Absorption leads to speedier setting times; evaporation slows it down. If sufficient evaporation has occurred for crystals to appear in the bottle the liquid *must be discarded*.

Copper Cements

USE

To cement splints to the teeth of patients with fractured jaws.

PROPERTIES

1. Similar to zinc phosphate cement, but the powder contains a copper compound in addition to zinc oxide. The colour varies according to the type of copper oxide:—

Red if cuprous oxide.

Black if cupric oxide.

2. Black cement is bactericidal.

3. Black cement has a worse effect on pulp than has the unmodified zinc oxyphosphate.

TECHNIQUE

Similar to oxyphosphate.

Glass–Ionomer (ASPA) Cement

ASPA relates to both silicates and polycarboxylates. It combines certain properties of both. The name is derived from Alumino Silicate PolyAcrylic acid.

USES

1. Erosion cavities.

2. Deciduous restorations.

3. Cementation of porcelain crowns.

4. Fissure Sealants.

PROPERTIES

1. Consists of a powder and liquid.

   Powder relates to silicates, consisting of fused quartz and alumina.

   Liquid consists of a 50 per cent solution of polyacrylic acid, stabilized to prevent gelling and thickening.

2. Has adhesive properties similar to zinc polycarboxylate cement.

3. As strong and translucent as silicates, i.e. superior to zinc oxide-based materials.

IDEAL IMPRESSION MATERIALS

These should:—

1. Be non-toxic

2. Be soft at temperatures which cause no harm or discomfort to the patient.

3. Record full details of the mouth and teeth.

4. Harden or set at mouth temperature.

5. Set in three to five minutes.

6. Remain dimensionally stable after removal from the mouth, or with storage.

The commonly used materials fall into three categories:—

Rigid, e.g., plaster-of-Paris.

Plastic, e.g., compositions, zinc oxide paste, waxes.

Elastic, e.g., alginates, rubber base, silicone rubbers.

PLASTER-OF-PARIS

The name originated during the Renaissance, when a good sculpture plaster was obtained from gypsum mined in Montmartre, Paris.

USES

1. Impressions, especially of edentulous mouths.
2. Models of teeth for reference purposes, and for construction of dentures, crowns, bridges, and orthodontic appliances.
3. In refractory investment materials used during the casting of inlays and crowns.

TECHNIQUE

Plaster is slowly sifted on to the surface of water contained in a bowl. This is continually tapped against the bench, causing water to be taken up by the powder and air-bubbles to be expelled. Plaster is added until no free water remains. Gentle spatulation produces a creamy mix. Rapid spatulation would incorporate air-bubbles which cause inaccuracies. Insufficient powder leads to delayed setting and weak plaster. If an impression breaks during removal from the mouth the pieces are re-joined with model cement (sticky wax).

HYDROCAL

Chemically similar to plaster-of-Paris, but differs physically. It is much stronger and harder, and is thus suitable for models.

Casting Models from Impressions: Impressions provide a negative picture of the dental structures. To construct a positive model, hydrocal or plaster-of-Paris is poured into the impression. It is gently mixed and slowly run into one side of the impression, gently vibrating the tray to ensure full contact between plaster and impression. Unless great care is taken at this time air-bubbles will be trapped, with loss of accuracy.

In the case of a plaster impression, a separating medium is applied before adding the model plaster, which would otherwise stick to it. Substances used are dilute water glass, colloidin varnish, and soap solution.

After the model has set the impression material is removed; plaster is chipped away, composition and zinc-oxide paste are heated, and the others are cut away. Finally the model is trimmed to ensure a neat finish.

IMPRESSION COMPOUNDS

Whereas plaster-of-Paris hardens by chemical means, compositions are thermoplastic. They soften with heat and harden upon cooling to mouth temperature. As this property is retained the material can be re-used.

Group 1

Little or no elasticity, so do not reproduce undercuts. Soften at 55–60° C.

Uses

1. Copper ring impressions for inlays and crowns.
2. Functional or compressive impressions for dentures.

Group 2

Sufficiently elastic to reproduce two-thirds of an undercut. Soften at 60–70° C.

Uses

Impressions of mouths with small undercuts.

Group 3

Relatively tough. Soften at 70° C.

Uses

Support for other materials, as special trays.

Technique

They are softened in hot water. Gauze or cloth around the inside of the bowl prevents the material from sticking to it. The composition should be thoroughly kneaded with the fingers. The softened material is placed in a warm dry tray and roughly shaped to the dental arch. The surface is then slightly Vaselined, passed through a flame to make it sufficiently soft, and an impression is taken. After cooling to mouth temperature it is removed and placed in cold water to harden it finally, thus reducing the possibility of distortion.

For crowns and inlays the softened composition is used in a copper ring instead of in an impression tray.

Plaster is poured directly into the composition, no separating medium being needed. Composition is removed from the model by softening in water at 65–70° C.

ZINC OXIDE AND EUGENOL IMPRESSION PASTES

These are not elastic and so do not accurately record undercuts. Setting is due to a chemical change instead of due to heat.

USES

1. Impression for relining full dentures. Used as a thin wash inside the denture, which is first cut away on the fitting surfaces.

2. Accurate impressions for full dentures are taken inside a preliminary composition impression, base plate of bite block, or old denture.

3. With wisps of cotton-wool as a periodontal pack.

TECHNIQUE

The material is supplied in two tubes, each usually containing different coloured pastes. Equal lengths of both are squeezed on to a waxed-paper pad. Little is required as the material is used only to a thickness of 1–2 mm. They are mixed with a broad-bladed spatula until the two colours combine as one. The material is very sticky and stings, so the patient's lips should be given a light coating of petroleum jelly; the nurse will also find it useful to smear some on her own fingers prior to mixing the paste.

No separating medium is required prior to casting.

GUTTA PERCHA

A thermoplastic and rubbery material.

USES

1. Impression for cleft palate plates (obturators).
2. Temporary denture relining material.
3. Temporary fillings.
4. Root-canal filling points (sterilized by storing in spirit).
5. Lining for tissue-borne (Gunning) splints.

ALGINATES (HYDROCOLLOIDS)

Many varieties may be purchased but all consist of powders to be mixed with water. It is most important to carry out the manufacturers' instructions carefully.

USES

Impressions for partial dentures, orthodontic appliances, and splints.

TECHNIQUE

A measured quantity of powder is spread on to the surface of a measured volume of water and the two are mixed to a homogenous paste. A long-bladed, flexible spatula, allows firm pressure against the side of the plastic or rubber bowl, in which mixing takes place.

Note: if the powder is left in a damp atmosphere it becomes wet and solidifies. Therefore *the packet must always be kept tightly closed.*

Retention in the tray is by using:
1. Perforated trays, some material passing through the holes to rivet the impression into position.
2. Molten sticky (yellow) wax.
3. Cotton-wool fibres stuck to the tray.
4. Quick-drying adhesive.
5. Elastoplast.

No separating medium is required prior to casting, which should ideally be carried out immediately. If this is not possible, the impression should be wrapped in a damp napkin and enclosed in a polythene bag to keep it moist. This prevents warpage. Alginate is removed from the model by cutting it away.

ELASTOMERS (RUBBER POLYMERS)

Two types of rubber-like polymers (elastomers) are used as impression materials.
1. Polysulphides (rubber base, Thiokol).
2. Silicones.

Uses

Impressions for crowns, bridges, inlays, and partial dentures where deep undercuts exist.

General Properties Elastomers

1. Viscosity varies with composition of material.
2. Very accurate for recording detail.
3. Little contraction with setting.
4. Very elastic, thus less chance of breakage when withdrawn from undercuts.
5. Tougher than alginates.
6. Non-toxic or poisonous.

Properties of Polysulphides

1. Supplied as two pastes.
   Base of polysulphide plus filler (colours it white).
   Accelerator of lead dioxide (brown), plus sulphur and oil.
2. May be obtained in a variety of viscosities:—
a. Light bodied for injection by syringe.
b. Heavy bodied for using in a tray.
3. May be obtained with a diluent, to produce a thinner viscosity at the chairside.
4. Odour of pastes containing lead dioxide is unpleasant.

PROPERTIES OF SILICONES
1. Sold as two pastes, or a paste and a liquid.
2. Viscosity varies with the material:—
a. Thin for syringe.
b. Putty-like for tray.

TECHNIQUE FOR ELASTOMERS
Usually mixed with a broad-bladed spatula on a waxed paper pad for about 45 seconds, until no streaks remain, in a similar way to zinc oxide–eugenol pastes. Rubber solution is used to hold the material in the tray. Patient's lips are coated with Vaseline.

INLAY WAX

This material is softened over a flame. It hardens at mouth temperature. This enables it to be carved accurately with fine margins in the mouth. Although hard enough for the wax pattern to be withdrawn from the cavity, it is sufficiently brittle to break rather than bend, thus preventing inaccuracy. The colour contrasts with the tooth tissues, and is usually blue.

USES
Accurate direct impressions for gold inlays and crowns.

DENTURE MATERIALS

Dentures consist of a base plus teeth and clasps (for retention).
Teeth: Acrylic, porcelain.
Clasps: Gold, stainless steel, chrome cobalt.
Bases: Acrylic, gold, stainless steel, chrome cobalt, vulcanite (seldom used now).

WAXES

Can all be softened by gently passing over a flame or through warm water.
1. Blue inlay wax (*see above*).
2. Red carding wax: for recording a bite.
3. Pink denture wax: denture base for try-ins, waxing-up dentures, and bite blocks.

4. Sheet casting wax: construction of cast metal dentures (i.e., used to form the shape of the denture prior to casting into metal such as gold).

5. Yellow sticky wax (model cement): to repair plaster impressions and models, attachment of alginates to trays, to hold together parts of a broken denture prior to and during repair. It is melted in a flame.

ABRASIVE AGENTS

These must be harder than the materials to be abraded or smoothed.

Diamond

Usually as a coating of dust on the surface of a metal disk, cone, or bur. If clogged with tooth debris it should be scrubbed with soap and water.

Tungsten Carbide

The hardest of metals, used either as a rough surface or for the cutting edges of burs, chisels, and other tools.

Carborundum

Used in mounted stones and wheels during crown preparations.

Emery

Abrasive coat on paper strips or disks.

Sand

Used as small sandpaper disks. Smoother than carborundum. Used for finishing crown preparations.

Pumice

Powdered volcanic rock.

USES

1. To polish acrylic dentures.
2. For cleaning tartar deposits from enamel, without harming the latter.
3. Used with glycerin or alcohol to polish amalgam fillings.

POLISHING AGENTS

These must be softer than the material to be polished.

Whiting (Precipitated Chalk)

For metals and plastics. Used with water.

Rouge

For the final polishing of gold.

Tripoli

A mild abrasive used for retaining a very smooth surface.

Toothpastes

Consist of precipitated chalk, salt, soap or detergent, flavouring, colouring agents, plus an active ingredient such as fluoride or a disinfectant.

FISSURE SEALANTS

These are materials used to occlude stagnation areas in pits, fissures, and anatomical defects, thus preventing the onset of caries. Many materials have been developed for this purpose, but more recent techniques tend to utilize resin systems that can be applied directly to the teeth.

It is too early to know how long sealants will stay on teeth, and whether or not they prove to be a major preventive agent.

THE IDEAL SEALANT

1. Relatively low viscosity, flowing easily into the depths of pits and fissures.
2. Capable of maintaining intimate contact with the tooth.
3. Resists occlusal wear.
4. Not soluble in saliva.
5. Bactericidal.
6. Easily and quickly applied.

AVAILABLE MATERIALS

1. Acrylic polymers.
2. Glass-ionomer cements.
3. Dimethacrylate polymers.
4. Cyanoacrylates.

Dimethacrylates

The two major products consist of methacrylate monomer and Bis-GMA. One is activated chemically, the other by ultra-violet light. Little difference has yet been shown between the various systems.

QUESTIONS

1. For what purposes and how are the following materials normally used in dentistry ?
   a. Inlay wax.
   b. Gutta percha.
   c. Impression paste.
   d. Impression compound.

2. What are the uses of silver amalgam and silicate cements ? Describe in detail the preparation of one of these substances for insertion in a cavity. How should waste amalgam be stored ?

3. Describe the preparation and method of use of three of the following impression materials. What precautions should be observed in each case until the models are cast ?
   a. Composition.
   b. Plaster.
   c. Alginate.
   d. Rubber base.

4. Compare and contrast zinc oxide–eugenol and oxyphosphate cements.

CHAPTER XII

OPERATIVE DENTAL SURGERY

RESTORATIVE DENTISTRY

THIS is the branch of dentistry concerned with the replacement of lost tooth tissue. It includes conservation and prosthetics.

Conservation: Restoration of tissue by means of fillings, inlays, crowns, and bridges.

Prosthetics: Restoration by full or partial dentures. Bridges are sometimes regarded as fixed prostheses.

Fillings

The objects of filling teeth are:—
1. Elimination of pain.
2. Attainment of maximum function and aesthetics.

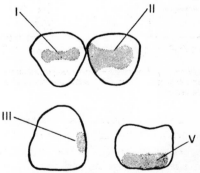

Fig. 39.—Classification of cavities and fillings. I, occlusal; II, proximal-occlusal in posteriors; III, proximal in anteriors; V, cervicals.

3. Preservation of health of the pulp.
4. Prevention of further caries.

Fillings are classified according to their position on teeth (*Fig.* 39).

CAVITY PREPARATION

The basic need is to eliminate caries from the tooth, to prevent its recurrence, and to ensure that the filling does not fall out. For descriptive purposes the process is described in several stages, but in practice these are all integrated.

Outline Form of the Cavity Margin: The cavity is cut through enamel to just reach the dentine layer, passing through all defective fissures until sound tooth substance is reached.

Extension for prevention involves:—

a. Enlarging the cavity so that the usual sites of stagnation and caries are eliminated.

b. Placing the margins of the cavity in such a position that edges of fillings can be readily cleaned by mastication and toothbrush. Further caries is thus less likely to occur.

It is therefore common practice to cut out all the fissures and to place the margins about one-third of the way up the cuspal slopes. In interproximal cavities the buccal and lingual margins are just visible from these aspects. The gingival margin must be out of contact with the adjoining tooth, below the contact point.

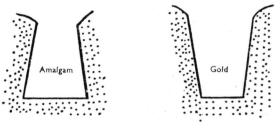

Fig. 40.–Diagram showing that cavities cut for amalgam converge occlusally to retain the filling material. Those for gold are shaped to allow withdrawal of the impression material.

Retention Form: This is a means of ensuring that fillings do not fall out. The side walls of the cavity are made slightly convergent occlusally (*Fig.* 40); alternatively an undercut is placed in the dentine layer. To prevent Class II fillings moving into the interproximal space, a lock is cut into the occlusal surface. Class V cavities are retained by occlusally and gingivally placed undercuts.

Removal of Remaining Caries: In many cases all decay has been removed during the above procedures. If not, the remainder is carefully removed with an excavator or round bur.

LININGS AND TEMPORARY DRESSINGS

During cavity preparation a large area of dentine is exposed. This and the pulp must be protected from damage by hot and cold foods by a lining material such as zinc oxide and eugenol or zinc oxyphosphate cement. A temporary dressing is placed in very deep cavities until the tooth has settled down and secondary dentine has formed to protect the pulp. A quick-setting zinc oxide and eugenol mixture is very suitable for this purpose.

AMALGAM FILLINGS

These are used to fill Class I, II, and V cavities in posterior teeth. After the amalgam filling is mixed it is picked up in a special carrier and handed to the dentist, who places it into the tooth cavity. He presses the amalgam into place with a hand or mechanical amalgam plugger, ensuring close adaptation to the cavity walls and bringing excess mercury to the surface. Carving removes excess amalgam and restores the tooth to its original anatomical form, this being best for maximum functional efficiency. Formation of a marginal ridge prevents food reaching and damaging the gingivae. Carving also attains a level joint between tooth enamel and amalgam. If this were not done food would catch in this region, stagnate, and lead to recurrent decay, as well as gingivitis if at gum level.

Twenty-four hours or longer after inserting the filling the surface is polished with amalgam finishing burs, abrasive strips and discs, brushes, pumice and glycerine, or zinc oxide in alcohol, to ensure a final smooth finish.

Summary of Requirements for Successful Amalgam Restorations:

1. Use the correct ratio of alloy and mercury according to the manufacturer's instructions (*see* Chapter X).

2. Careful and thorough trituration.

3. Immediately pack into cavity.

4. Condense with heavy pressure to ensure the removal of excess mercury.

5. Carve to the correct anatomical form.

6. Polish to ensure a smooth surface, with no edges between tooth and amalgam.

Matrix Bands: Whereas it is quite simple to pack amalgam into a simple Class I cavity, it is not so easy to do this in a Class II. When amalgam is placed in such a cavity it falls out into the interproximal region. A matrix band placed around the tooth replaces any missing wall and prevents filling material leaving the cavity, even with maximum condensing pressure. Various types of matrix holders and bands may be obtained (each with a different use).

The correct band is positioned around the tooth and a wedge is placed between this band and the next tooth. This holds the matrix band firmly against the neck of the tooth to be filled, which ensures correct adaptation of the filling cervically, and prevents formation of an amalgam ledge with subsequent gingival irritation.

Armamentarium required for Amalgam Fillings:
Diagnostic kit—mirror, probe, tweezers.
Handpiece and burs.
Excavators and chisels.
Amalgam pluggers.
Plastic instruments.
Amalgam carvers.
Matrix holders and bands.
Wedges.
Saliva ejector.
Chip syringe.
Amalgamator or pestle and mortar.

SILICATE FILLINGS

Silicates are used to fill Class III and Class V cavities, and to face gold inlays in anterior teeth. Although aesthetically superior, they only tend to last three or four years.

Whenever possible a rubber dam is applied to the tooth prior to inserting a silicate filling, as the latter is weakened and discoloured in the presence of moisture. A lining is always placed over exposed dentine to prevent free acid in the silicate cement from irritating the pulp.

For silicates the matrix takes the form of a celluloid strip, which may be held in position with a special clamp. Silicate is placed into the cavity with a plastic instrument and a strip lightly smeared with petroleum jelly is used to compress it tightly into position. After the filling has set hard the strip is easily removed, the petroleum jelly acting as a separating medium. Excess material is removed with a scalpel blade and white stones smeared with petroleum jelly, and a coating of varnish is applied. This stops uptake of moisture and stains before the final set has taken place. After twenty-four hours the filling is polished with fine stones, disks, and strips, all greased with petroleum jelly.

Armamentarium for Silicate Fillings: In addition to those required for amalgam fillings:—
Shade guide.
Celluloid strips.
Petroleum jelly.
Surface varnish.
Agate or stellite spatula.
Glass slab.

Automatic mixer, if used.
Rubber dam, clamps, forceps, punch, frame.
Silk floss.

ACRYLIC RESIN

This has been used in the past but due to its poor physical properties it is now seldom utilized. It tends to shrink and rapidly discolour. Acrylic consists of a liquid and powder which are mixed together at the chairside, and is inserted in a manner similar to that described for silicate cements.

COMPOSITES

These are used for Class III and V fillings, and for restoring fractured incisors. Prior to filling, the cavity is lined, but not with zinc oxide–eugenol, as this stains composite and inhibits its setting reaction. Enamel around the edge of the cavity is etched with a 50 per cent solution of phosphoric acid, to aid retention.

Composite is packed into the cavity with a plastic spatula and a polythene matrix band or crown former is used to hold the material firmly in place for about two minutes. The matrix is then removed, and excess material is cut away with a sharp blade.

Ideally, no further excess should remain, but if necessary further material can be removed after six minutes. Diamonds, carbide finishing burs, green stones and zirconium strips are all used. Final finishing is done with fine silicone carbide paper-backed discs and white Arkansas stones, using water or a special lubricant.

Armamentarium for Composite Fillings:
Shade guide.
Composite kit.
Polythene matrices and crown formers.
Plastic spatula.
Sharp knife.
Finishing discs, stones, etc.
Lubricant.

Badly Broken-down Teeth

These require more complex means of restoring lost tooth tissue. Sometimes amalgam can still be used; in order to increase its retention small holes are cut in the tooth and pins or screws placed into them. Amalgam is then built up around these aids to retention. In order to allow the amalgam to set properly before final shaping, the patient is occasionally sent away with the matrix band still in place. A copper ring modified to the tooth and gingival contour may be used for this purpose.

In situations where amalgam is not strong enough, gold or stainless-steel crowns are used, the former being the most common. Porcelain and acrylic crowns are used for the restoration of anterior teeth.

GOLD INLAYS AND CROWNS

Gold provides a very strong and durable means of restoring a tooth. It is cast outside the mouth to fit the prepared tooth accurately. Inlays and crowns are used to restore teeth where much tooth tissue has been lost.

The preparation of a tooth to receive a gold inlay is similar to that involved for amalgam fillings, except that in this case no undercuts are allowed (*see Fig.* 40). The walls are made to diverge slightly occlusally, making removal of the impression possible.

After the dentist has prepared and lined the cavity he takes an impression or pattern, so that his technician can construct a gold inlay to fit the tooth. Indirect and direct techniques may be used. In the latter case a wax pattern is constructed on the tooth itself and then taken away to be processed by the technician. With the indirect technique an accurate model of the patient's tooth is constructed from an impression and the wax prepared on this. In both cases the inlay is later cemented into the tooth.

Direct Technique: Blue inlay wax is gently softened by warming and pressed into the cavity. After cooling to mouth temperature, the surface is carved with a wax carver, and smoothed with cotton-wool and hot water. A metal sprue is added to aid removal of the wax pattern from the tooth and the pattern is sent to a laboratory technician. He embeds the wax impression in a refractory material (similar to plaster). This is then heated to melt the wax, the gaseous remnants of which evaporate through the sprue hole, leaving behind a cavity or mould. Molten gold is forced into this by a process of casting. After cooling, the gold is cleaned, the non-fitting surfaces are polished, and the inlay is returned to the dentist.

Indirect Technique: An impression is taken of the prepared cavity using a copper ring filled with warm composition, or a tray containing rubber base or one of the elastic impression materials. The dentist also takes an impression of the opposing teeth, and the patient is asked to bite into a piece of softened pink wax to record the bite. This enables the technician to know how thick to make the occlusal portion of gold.

From these impressions the technician makes a set of models on which he then constructs the inlay, using techniques similar to those for the direct technique.

Copper Ring Technique: The correct size of copper ring is adapted to the shape of tooth and gingivae with crown scissors. The ring is filled with warm composition and pressed against the tooth until the material hardens, providing an impression of the cut tooth surface. In order to show the technician the relationship between the tooth in question and those on either side, a localizing impression is taken, using rubber base, silicone rubber, or plaster-of-Paris in a bridge tray.

The surgery assistant must carefully pack the impression in a box so that there is no distortion, chipping, or loss on the way to the technician. The names of patient and dentist should be enclosed, together with any necessary instructions to the technician.

Armamentarium for Copper Ring Impressions:
Selection of copper rings.
Crown scissors.
Bunsen or spirit-lamp flame.
Composition and silicone rubber.
Petroleum jelly.
Bridge and other trays.
Pink bite-wax.

TEMPORARY COVER

This is placed on any tooth prepared for a crown or inlay until the final restoration is ready.

1. It prevents pain due to food and air acting on exposed dentine.

2. It stops the teeth on each side and in occlusion from drifting towards the prepared tooth, into the space previously occupied by the tooth tissue which has just been removed, i.e., it occupies the space which will later be filled by the final restoration.

Suitable temporary materials are quick-setting zinc oxide and eugenol (possibly mixed with cotton-wool), aluminium crowns, copper rings, and celluloid crown formers (anterior teeth only).

CROWNS

These are constructed to resemble the natural teeth in shape and colour. Gold, porcelain, and acrylic are used, the first in sites where strength is the foremost requirement, and the others where aesthetics are more important. Stainless steel is sometimes used for deciduous teeth and for temporary crowns on fractured permanent teeth. As with inlays there are three clinical phases of construction, involving two visits to the surgery.

1. Preparation of the tooth.
2. Impression taking.
3. Fitting of the restoration.

Jacket Crowns: These are made to cap anterior teeth which are so badly damaged by decay that normal fillings are no longer possible. They are also used to improve the the appearance of hypoplastic, discoloured, fractured, and displaced teeth.

Tooth tissue is cut away so as to leave a core of dentine. Impressions and bite are taken using techniques similar to those described for gold inlays, and a temporary crown is placed in position. The shade or colour of the nearby teeth is recorded. The technician then constructs a crown, which is cemented on to the tooth with a thin mix of oxyphosphate cement.

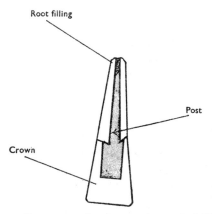

Fig. 41.—Post crown showing previous apical filling.

Post Crowns: With extensive destruction of tooth tissue it is no longer possible to retain a jacket crown. Under these circumstances a post crown is constructed. Most of the remaining part of the erupted tooth is cut away and a hole is drilled in the root canal for about two-thirds of its length. It is therefore necessary to first extirpate the pulp and place a root filling in the apical one-third of the canal. Then an impression is taken of the inside of the canal and a gold post is made to fit this. The top part of the post is built up to resemble a tooth stump prepared for a jacket crown, and an acrylic or porcelain crown is fitted over this core (*Fig.* 41). In some cases pre-formed posts are purchased and adapted at the chairside.

Stainless-steel Crowns: These are used to restore badly broken down deciduous molars, and as temporary covers on fractured permanent incisors. Caries is removed and the dentine is covered with a zinc-oxide cement. All undercuts are ground away with green stones or diamond cutters, and the occlusal surface is taken out of contact with the opposing tooth so as to allow a thickness of metal to be placed later in that position. A stainless-steel crown of the requisite size is adapted to the gingival margin with crown scissors and pliers, and is then cemented into position.

Endodontic Therapy

This is treatment of the pulp, and includes root filling, pulpotomy, and pulp capping.

Root-canal Therapy

Chemical, thermal, and bacterial irritants lead to inflammation and necrosis of the pulp. Thus this occurs below unlined silicate fillings and deep caries, and after over-heating during cavity preparation; cold water is therefore sprayed on teeth when cutting with high-speed instruments. In the event of pulpal pathology the tissue is removed or extirpated (pulpectomy) and the resultant space is filled with a root-canal filling.

If the pulp is vital a local anaesthetic is administered. A saliva ejector is placed in the mouth and a rubber dam positioned over the tooth in question to isolate it from the oral cavity with its multitudes of bacteria. A hole is made in the rubber dam with a punch. The dam is held in place with clamps or silk floss and spread out over a frame. The tooth is swabbed with an antiseptic such as tincture of iodine to sterilize its surface and the operation is commenced.

All instruments used in endodontic therapy must be absolutely sterile. In some practices they are made up as sterile root-canal kits and kept in readiness for use when required. A small electric glass bead or other type of sterilizer may be kept at the chairside to re-sterilize small instruments during the operation. In order to keep the canal free from bacteria it is essential for the dentist to work as speedily as possible so that the canal is only open to the air for a minimum period of time. It is therefore most important for his surgery assistant to have everything ready as and when required.

Entry to the pulp chamber is made with a bur, and the pulp is removed with a barbed broach. The canal is cleaned with mechanical reamers and files of ascending size until healthy firm dentine is reached.

The canal is then washed with sterile water, or alternate applications of hydrogen peroxide and Milton. It is dried with cotton-wool pellets and paper points. An antiseptic such as parachlorphenol is inserted on a paper point, or a mixture of antibiotics is spun in with a rotary paste filler. The dressing is sealed in with cotton-wool, and then zinc oxide and eugenol.

If required a check may be made of the organisms present in the canal. After washing it out, a paper point is placed into the canal close to the apex, for one minute. It is then placed in a culture tube containing a special medium and sent to a laboratory for bacteriological examination. A report is later returned to the dentist outlining the organisms present and the drugs which should be used to eradicate them from the canal.

At the next visit the tooth is again isolated and the canal re-opened. The dressing is removed and the canal is re-reamed, washed, dried, and dressed. This procedure is repeated at weekly intervals until the tooth is free from infection, as judged from lack of signs and symptoms of inflammation, and from absence of organisms in the culture.

Root-canal Fillings: In order to prevent further entry of organisms into the canal it is filled with a gutta percha or silver point. This is placed so as to just reach the root apex, being neither short nor projecting through into the surrounding tissues. Either of these faults could give rise to further inflammation.

To ensure that the point is placed at the apex, the length of the canal is calculated. A reamer or smooth broach of known length is placed into the canal and a radiograph is taken. The apparent length as shown on the resulting X-ray picture is measured and the true length of canal is calculated from the following formula, everything else being known.

$$\frac{\text{True length of canal}}{\text{X-ray length of canal}} = \frac{\text{True length of reamer}}{\text{X-ray length of reamer}}$$

A point of the required length is then cemented into position in the canal with quick-setting zinc oxide and eugenol or a root-canal sealing cement (*Fig.* 42).

Armamentarium for Root-canal Therapy:
Mirror, probe, and tweezers.
Rubber dam, frame, clamps, punch, and forceps.
Silk floss.
Saliva ejector.
Handpiece and burs.
Reamers and files.
Broaches, plain and barbed.

Cotton-wool pellets.
Paper points.
Excavators and plastic instruments.
Syringe with sterile water.
Hydrogen peroxide and Milton.
Antiseptic such as parachlorphenol.
Polyantibiotic paste.
Rotary paste filler.
Root-canal cement.
Gutta-percha or silver points.

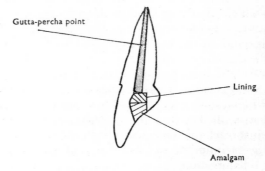

Gutta-percha point

Lining

Amalgam

Fig. 42.—A typical root filling.

PULPOTOMY

Removal of only part of the pulp, usually that section within the crown, leaving vital pulp tissue in the root canals. This operation is performed on a young permanent incisor tooth when the pulp has been exposed traumatically during cavity preparation or by a blow that has fractured the crown. In such a tooth the root is not fully formed, the pulp canal being very wide and the apex funnel-shaped. This would make root-canal filling very difficult. The operator therefore removes that part of the pulp which may be infected but leaves the healthy portion. The root therefore continues to form in the usual way. This procedure is sometimes carried out on a posterior tooth in which root-canal therapy is impossible because of the shape of the root canals.

After giving a local anaesthetic the tooth is isolated with rubber dam and its surface is sterilized. The coronal pulp is exposed further and then removed with a large round bur or an excavator. When bleeding stops, the stump is covered with a sterile mixture of calcium hydroxide powder and water. Over this is placed a lining of quick-setting zinc oxide and eugenol, and then an amalgam filling.

Pulp Capping

A means of protecting the pulp by covering small non-infected exposures with calcium hydroxide, over which is placed a small, firm celluloid or metal pulp cap, followed by a lining and an amalgam filling. Calcium hydroxide stimulates the formation of protective secondary dentine over the wound. Pulp caps prevent the transmission of pressure to exposed pulps.

Dentures

These may be classified according to whether they replace some or all teeth, and whether masticatory and other pressures are borne by the teeth or by bone and oral mucosa:—

1. Tissue-borne.
2. Tooth-borne.
3. Tooth-and-tissue-borne (load shared between teeth and surrounding tissues).

As full dentures restore jaws in which no natural teeth remain, they are always tissue-borne. However, partial dentures may fall into any of the above categories. When supported by the teeth alone they may be fixed permanently to these, or they may be removable from the mouth. In the former case they are known as *bridges*.

Full Dentures

These consist of a full set of artificial teeth embedded in a base. Teeth are constructed of acrylic or porcelain. Acrylic, stainless steel, gold, and (rarely) vulcanite are used for denture base construction.

There are four clinical stages in the construction of dentures:—

1. Impressions.
2. Taking the bite.
3. Try-in.
4. Final fitting.

Impressions: A means of reproducing the shape of the patient's jaws in the laboratory so that a technician can construct an accurately fitting denture. Impression materials are more fully discussed in Chapter XI.

The selected material is placed in an impression tray and kept in the patient's mouth for the required length of time, according to the material being used. If no available tray accurately fits the dental arches, a provisional impression is taken, usually with composition, and a special tray is constructed in the laboratory. This enables a more accurate impression to be taken later.

Impressions should either be cast immediately, or be well packed to prevent damage and dehydration during their journey to the laboratory.

Bites: The dentist must indicate to his technician the relationship which exists between the patient's dental arches. For this a 'bite' is taken. The technician can later place the plaster models into the bite blocks, thus reproducing the same relationships as exists between the jaws. For the edentulous patient special wax bite blocks are constructed. In addition to their recording both the vertical and antero-posterior relationship between the jaws, the dentist marks on them the position of the lips, the corners of the mouth, and the facial midline. At the same time a shade is recorded.

Try-in: The technician sets up the teeth in a wax base, which is returned to the dentist for trying in the patient's mouth. Modifications are easily made at this stage, until both patient and dentist are satisfied as to fit, comfort, aesthetics, and masticatory efficiency.

Fitting the Dentures: The technician processes the try-in so as to replace the wax base by an acrylic resin. The finished product is returned to the dentist for fitting in the patient's mouth.

After any necessary adjustments the patient receives instructions on how to clean the denture and is then allowed to go away. He is asked to return a few days later to check that all is well. Under no circumstances should he attempt to make any adjustments himself. The dentures should be washed with a toothbrush and paste whilst being held over a bowl of water. This prevents fracture of the denture if it is dropped at any time. When left out of the mouth dentures should be kept in water to prevent distortion. Ideally, they should not be worn at night to give the oral tissues a rest.

PARTIAL DENTURES

These are very similar to full dentures except that they are placed where some natural teeth remain. Retention is aided by clasps, which are metal projections that grip the remaining teeth. The tooth-bearing areas are known as 'saddles'.

Impressions for these are taken in box trays. For the ' bite ' a small piece of softened wax or elastic impression material is placed in the mouth, and the patient is asked to close his teeth into it. The technician can later place the model teeth into the marks thus made.

BRIDGES

These consist of one or more artifical teeth embedded in an acrylic base. They may be fixed to one or more of the remaining teeth, but are occasionally removable. Prior to their construction the teeth on which they rest have to be prepared, frequently as inlay or crown preparations.

The impression and laboratory phases are similar to those for partial dentures.

QUESTIONS

1. Describe the following and briefly indicate the circumstances in which they may be used:—
   a. Copper band.
   b. Alginate impression material.
   c. Modelling wax (pink).
   d. Stainless-steel wire.

2. Describe the instruments and materials which may be required at the various stages of root-canal treatment in connexion with an upper permanent incisor tooth.

3. What are the stages in the construction of full dentures ? What parts do the dental surgeon and surgery assistant each play ?

4. What instruments and materials would be required to trim and polish:—
   a. A large two-surface amalgam filling ?
   b. A silicate filling ?
   c. A gold inlay ?

CHAPTER XIII

MINOR ORAL SURGERY AND PERIODONTAL THERAPY

ASEPSIS PRIOR TO MINOR ORAL SURGERY

TRUE surgical asepsis is not possible in the mouth, as it contains a multitude of bacterial organisms. Some of these are harmful, others less so. Most important is the reduction of oral organisms, and no introduction of fresh ones from outside sources.

It is therefore important that all patients for surgery have a clean mouth. Poor oral hygiene carries a high risk of infection at the site of operation.

The use of sterile gloves, gowns, instruments, and dressings will minimize the risk of sepsis. The dental surgery assistant thus holds a position of special responsibility where sterility is concerned. She can contribute a great deal towards both the well-being of the patients and the high reputation and standard of the practice.

CLEANING OF HANDS

Hands and nails should be thoroughly scrubbed immediately prior to any operation. Whenever possible sterile disposable gloves should be worn, as they minimize all risk of the transfer of organisms. They should be thrown away after use.

DRESSINGS

These are best sterilized by autoclaving. Pre-sterilized packs can sometimes be obtained from a local hospital with a Central Sterilization Department. This saves time and worry.

INSTRUMENTS

Instruments must be thoroughly sterilized (*see* Chapter VII) and laid under a sterile cloth, and not touched afterwards except with sterile gloves.

They should be placed in the required order on a sterile towel, within easy reach of the operator. The choice of instruments varies according to the individual surgeon's preference. Always lay them out in the same order so that they can quickly be found. Very sharp-edged instruments such as chisels and scalpels should be placed carefully on their sides on sterile lint or similar material to prevent any risk of blunting the cutting edges.

After use they should be placed in a sterilized dish, so that they are available for re-use if required, without contaminating other instruments which have not been used.

PREPARATION OF PATIENT FOR SURGERY

One of the most important aspects is the psychological preparation of the patient by helping to allay any fears. A well-groomed and informed dental surgery assistant can be very helpful at this stage. She should be able to explain the procedure in simple language, using terms that the patient can understand without becoming frightened. This produces far more satisfactory results than any drug. If necessary, the dentist may give a sedative either for use the night before, or for immediately before the operation. The former will help the patient to have a good night's rest.

The dental surgery assistant must ensure that a patient receives the correct instructions for preparation for an operation, and that these are carried out. Nervous people do not always comprehend everything said to them, so make certain that instructions are given clearly, and even written down if necessary.

The patient should arrive at the surgery about 15 minutes before treatment to allow him to settle down before the operation.

If local anaesthesia is to be used, ensure that the patient understands the importance of having a meal before coming to the surgery, and explain that this will prevent nausea and fainting. If they fail to eat, a drink of glucose can be given at the surgery.

If a general anaesthetic is to be administered, explain that the patient must not eat nor drink for at least four hours beforehand. On arrival he should empty his bladder, loosen any tight clothing, and remove any artificial dentures.

Seat the patient in the dental chair so as to provide maximum comfort for both him and the dentist. Place a sterile towel around his neck. A bright smile and encouraging words at this stage can do much to alleviate any tension.

THE OPERATION

The patient's records and X-rays should be on hand, for easy reference throughout the operation. The surgery assistant should be sufficiently aware of what is going on surgically so as to be of intelligent assistance to the dentist throughout the operation. A surgeon must clearly see his field of work all the time, so his surgery assistant should yield an efficient aspirator to suck away blood, saliva, and debris. She should also hand him any necessary instruments.

POSTOPERATIVE CARE

When the operation has been completed, the patient should rest until fit to go home. During this time he must not be allowed to disturb other patients in the surgery or waiting room. This cannot be too strongly emphasized. A well conducted surgery makes suitable arrangements for the comfort of patients both before and after treatment without disturbing the smooth running of the practice. Children should be given every care and attention to prevent any future anxiety concerning visits to the dentist.

CONSENT FOR TREATMENT

No treatment may be carried out for any patient without his approval, which should be obtained in writing. In the case of minors below the age of 16 years the consent of a parent or guardian is required. Otherwise any treatment given may be regarded as an act of assault.

EXTRACTIONS

INDICATIONS
1. Orthodontics—to relieve crowding.
2. Gross decay.
3. Gross periodontal involvement.
4. Impaction, especially of mandibular third molars.
5. Pericoronitis due to a tooth continually biting on a gum flap.

TECHNIQUE

Teeth are removed by gripping the crown or root with forceps, and levering gently bucally and lingually to enlarge the socket. Sometimes an elevator is used. This is placed between the tooth and its proximal partner, and then gently rotated. This raises the tooth from within its socket. Sometimes the latter is first enlarged and the periodontal fibres cut by means of a Coupland's chisel.

Removal of Roots and Buried Teeth

Retained roots are encountered as a complication of an extraction being performed at the time, or as a result of breakage at some earlier date. Removal of roots is a planned procedure. Unless fully in view, extraction is only carried out after careful clinical and radiographic assessment. From this the root shape and position can be seen, as can any associated pathology and the density of the surrounding bone. Buried roots are uncovered by cutting a flap and removing bone.

The principles involved in removing unerupted teeth are exactly the same. Sometimes it is first necessary to divide the crown from the root in order to ease removal.

Raising a Flap

In edentulous regions a scalpel incision is normally made slightly lingual to the alveolar ridge. Anteriorly it is then carried into the buccal sulcus, carefully avoiding any nerves or blood vessels in the area. If other teeth are adjacent to the root the incision is usually carried around the necks of these teeth. The flap of mucosa is then pulled away from the underlying bone with a periosteal elevator. If the root cannot be removed at this stage because it is being mechanically held in place by overlying bone, some of the latter is cut away with chisels or burs. The root is then removed with an elevator or forceps. The socket is cleaned with sterile saline solution and the flap is replaced and sutured into position.

Third Molars and Pericoronitis

The 'wisdom teeth' are the last to form. Sometimes there is insufficient room for them to erupt, especially in the mandible. This causes impaction against the tooth in front or against bone. A flap of mucosa sometimes remains, partly lying across the tooth surface. Food stagnates around partially erupted teeth, especially if there is a gum flap, leading to caries, gingivitis, and pericoronitis. In the latter case, an antiseptic such as gentian violet is painted on the flap and the patient is instructed to use hot saline mouth-baths. Any opposing tooth biting on the flap is ground out of occlusion or even extracted, and if infection is severe an antibiotic is administered. If the flap does not go away, it may be excised. Sometimes the impacted tooth is removed.

REMOVAL OF IMPACTED TEETH

Extraction sometimes proves to be a difficult and traumatic procedure, depending on the direction and degree of impaction. The latter is classified for convenience as soft tissue or boney tissue. With soft-tissue impaction the crown is covered only by mucosa, and at least part of the crown is usually erupted into the mouth. This type of case is particularly liable to develop pericoronitis.

As there is normally insufficient space for direct removal, it is necessary to first remove bone, and then divide crown and roots prior to their separate extraction. If much trauma is involved the patient may later experience pain and swelling.

APICECTOMY

It is sometimes impossible to eradicate infection completely from around the root apex of a non-vital tooth, even after a root filling has been placed into the previously sterilized root canal. In such circumstances one reflects a flap, cuts away some bone from over the root, and then cuts off the root apex. This is because the apical portion of the root often has lateral canals which cannot be sterilized. The canal entrance is then sealed with gutta percha, silver, or amalgam. At the same time the bone is curetted to remove any chronic abscess material. The area is washed with sterile saline solution, and the flap is sutured into position. A check radiograph is usually taken at this point.

CYSTS

Simple Apical Cysts

Appear on radiographs as circular dark areas around the root apex, surrounded by a thin white line which is continuous with the lamina dura lining the tooth socket. The tooth is always non-vital. Treatment is by extirpation of the pulp followed by root-canal filling. Apicectomy and enucleation (shelling out) of the cyst lining may be necessary.

Marsupialization of Large Cysts

Because of their large size and position some cysts cannot be removed by simple enucleation. Instead, the buccal or lingual cyst wall is removed and the cavity is left open to relieve pressure exerted by the cyst contents and to permit gradual reduction in size. Gauze soaked in a sedative solution such as Whitehead's varnish is often placed in the cavity to keep it open. The space slowly heals from below upwards. With this technique there is minimal trauma and treatment is very speedy, making it very suitable for old and ill patients. There is also less danger of damaging nearby structures, nerves, blood-vessels, and antral lining.

Dentigerous Cysts

Cysts around the crowns of partially or non-erupted *vital* teeth. In such cases the overlying lining is removed and the opening kept patent until the tooth erupts into its normal position.

SURGICAL PREPARATION OF THE MOUTH FOR DENTURES

The shape of bone and mucosa is sometimes modified to accommodate dentures that will provide maximum comfort and function.

Alveolectomy

Removal of some alveolar bone in order to eliminate large undercuts or sharp edges. After reflecting a flap, bone is removed with bone forceps, chisels, burs, and files.

Alveolotomy

In this case the bony septa within the sockets are removed and the buccal and lingual walls are then squeezed together. This enables the artificial teeth to be placed more palatally than were their natural predecessors, which helps them to look less protrusive. This is especially useful in gross skeletal Class II cases.

Fraenectomy

A large fraenum occasionally tends to displace dentures, especially in the upper jaw. In such cases the lip is gently pulled away from the alveolar ridge to define the fraenum. This is then cut away, and the remaining mucosa on either side is sutured together.

INSTRUMENTS REQUIRED FOR SURGICAL PROCEDURES

Extraction forceps.
Coupland's and other bone chisels.
Dental elevators.
Scalpel and blades.
Periosteal elevators.
Handpiece and burs.
Suture thread and needles.
Scissors.

POSTOPERATIVE CARE OF THE PATIENT

a. Instructions

After extractions the patient is instructed not to rinse his mouth for twelve hours to avoid disturbing the blood-clot. However, if an abscess was present the patient is told to use hot salt mouth rinses.

He can eat and drink normally but should try to avoid the extraction site. If bleeding recurs he should bite for ten minutes on a clean handkerchief previously soaked in hot water and then wrung out. If it still does not stop he should return to the dentist.

If pain is experienced after the injection wears off, the patient should take a proprietary analgesic tablet. If this does not help he should seek the advice of his dentist.

b. Control of Infection

The patient should rinse his mouth with hot salt water, starting twelve hours after the extraction. One teaspoonful of salt should be dissolved in a glass of hot water. This mouthbath is used every two hours, especially after meals. It should be continued for ten days.

After difficult extractions and traumatic surgery, or in the presence of much infection, the patient may be put on a course of antibiotic therapy.

c. Removal of Sutures

The patient should be given an appointment to return in about four days for the removal of stitches. At this time the sutures are gripped with tweezers or dissecting forceps, cut with fine scissors and gently withdrawn from the tissue.

HAEMOSTASIS OR CONTROL OF BLEEDING

Excessive haemorrhage may occur at the time of operation, or later, when it is secondary to some other factor such as mechanical disturbance of the clot, or infection.

Treatment of Primary Haemorrhage

If bleeding does not stop spontaneously within four minutes of the operation mechanical measures are taken. The socket is covered with a clean damp gauze and the patient is asked to gently bite upon this for ten minutes. If this is not successful the edges of the wound are drawn together and sutured, possibly first inserting a chemical haemostat agent such as viper venom or gelatin foam.

(For DELAYED OR SECONDARY HAEMORRHAGE, see Chapter XIV.)

ORO-ANTRAL FISTULA

As the roots of maxillary molars and premolars are so closely related to the floor and lining of the maxillary antrum, these are sometimes torn during tooth extraction. There is then direct continuity between the mouth and antrum. If left open this oro-antral fistula would allow passage of bacteria from the oral cavity to the sinus, leading to sinusitis or inflammation of the antrum.

It is therefore imperative to close the hole as speedily as possible, by pulling buccal and lingual mucosa across the opening and suturing them together.

MARGINAL GINGIVITIS

This must be treated early or the inflammation will spread to the periodontal membrane and bone. The early stages are treated by removal of the gingival irritant. The teeth are scaled to remove calculus, and then polished to smooth any roughened areas. The patient is taught how and when to clean his teeth and gums. This removes plaque and food debris and stimulates the gums, increasing their resistance to further infection.

Scaling

Mechanical removal of calculus from the tooth surface. The type of scaler used varies according to the site from which calculus is being removed.

Elimination of Other Causes of Gingivitis

Badly placed fillings, faulty dentures and orthodontic appliances, caries, and any other factors holding food in contact with the gingivae must be eliminated.

CHRONIC PERIODONTITIS

Careful treatment will prevent or at least delay further destruction of the periodontium with subsequent formation of true pockets. It involves the utmost co-operation by the patient. Treatment is directed towards:—

1. Removal of supra- and subgingival calculus and plaque, by scaling and polishing.
2. Elimination of stagnation areas due to poor fillings, dentures, etc.
3. Removal of pockets by gingivectomy.
4. Instruction of the patient in careful brushing of teeth and gums, and the use of wood points to cleanse and stimulate the interdental areas.

Gingivectomy

The removal of gingival tissue to eliminate pockets from around the teeth. It is only carried out after careful scaling and polishing has reduced the gingival irritation, so that the true depth of the remaining pocket can be evaluated.

Gingivectomy may also be used to remove pseudo-pockets associated with, for example, chronic hyperplasia due to Epanutin (phenytoin).

Gingivoplasty

Modified removal of tissue to restore the gingival contour, for example, in regions where the interdental papilla has been destroyed by an attack of acute ulcerative gingivitis.

Both gingivectomy and gingivoplasty can be carried out by use of surgical knives, chemicals, or electrocautery. The first is most commonly used.

PROCEDURE FOR SURGICAL GINGIVECTOMY

The patient is prepared for surgery in the usual way, and a local anaesthetic is administered. The depth of the pocket is measured with a pocket-measuring probe and the excess gingival tissue is marked with pocket-marking forceps. This excess tissue is then removed, including the portion lying between the teeth. After removing any remaining calculus from the area a dressing is placed over the raw surface to allow it to heal without being continually disturbed by food. Such a dressing may consist of zinc oxide and eugenol as a base, a hardener, and an antiseptic or an antibiotic. It is kept in place with cotton-wool strips pushed through interdental spaces. The dressing is removed after one week.

From that time on the patient must use wood points to keep the interdental spaces clean and to massage any remaining gum tissue. He must maintain careful toothbrushing habits. Immediately after operation a soft toothbrush is used, but later a harder one is substituted.

ARMAMENTARIUM FOR GINGIVECTOMY

Mirror, probe, tweezers.
Local anaesthetic and syringe.
Sucker.
Set of scaling instruments.
Periodontal hoes.
Curettes.
Periosteal elevator.
Gingivectomy knives.
Tissue forceps.
Pocket-marking forceps.
Probes.
Pocket-measuring probes.
Glass slab and spatula.
Forceps.
Fine scissors.
Gingivectomy pack.

PERIODONTAL ABSCESS

The abscess is drained and any infected tissue is removed by subgingival curettage. For this the bone and tooth surface are scraped to remove necrotic remains. Blood is left to fill the remaining space. In this way one hopes to obtain re-attachment between tooth and bone.

If access to deeper tissues is not possible by direct means, a gingival flap is cut and retracted to expose the underlying bone and root area.

Infected material, calculus, and superficial cementum are removed, and the raw mucosa is replaced almost in contact with the root surface, being only separated by blood-clot.

ACUTE ULCERATIVE GINGIVITIS (VINCENT'S DISEASE)

The first essential is relief of pain. Infected material is gently removed from the gum margin with cotton-wool and tweezers. Hydrogen peroxide is placed in the gingival crevices. As oxygen bubbles are released they provide an unfavourable environment for anaerobic bacteria as well as mechanically displacing any debris from this region. The patient may be given a hydrogen peroxide mouthwash for use at home. If he has an elevated temperature indicative of a generalized septicaemia an antibiotic such as penicillin is often administered.

The patient returns each day, and by the second or third day scaling is commenced to remove local irritation. After abatement of the acute phase gingivoplasty may be necessary. A strict regimen of maximum oral care must be imposed.

APHTHOUS ULCERS AND HERPETIC STOMATITIS

In both these conditions the treatment is symptomatic, providing maximum relief from pain and helping to prevent secondary infection by the use of antiseptic mouthbaths. If much pain is being experienced the patient is advised to eat soft foods such as soup and ice-cream.

QUESTIONS

1. In an operation for the extraction of an impacted lower third molar under local anaesthesia:—

   a. What preoperative instructions would the dental surgeon give to the patient ?

   b. What instruments and materials would you prepare ? State their uses.

2. What operative procedures may be undertaken for the prevention and treatment of periodontal disease ? What special instruments and materials would you provide for the operation of gingivectomy ?

3. Describe briefly the assistance which you could give to the dental surgeon in the following cases:—

   a. A patient suffering from a fainting attack.

   b. A refractory child.

   c. Persistent bleeding after extraction.

4. Briefly discuss:—
 a. Plaque control.
 b. Apicectomy.
 c. Pericoronitis.

CHAPTER XIV

DENTAL EMERGENCIES

IN this chapter we present a short resumé of some of the reasons for patients attending without appointments, usually in pain. Such dental emergencies require emergency treatment. An outline of such treatment is given below, except for those conditions dealt with in the preceding chapter.

OCCASIONAL TOOTHACHE

Usually starts when eating hot, cold, sweet, or sour foods, or when food is caught between two adjacent teeth. Debris and decay are removed and a quick-setting dressing is placed in the cavity, as a sedative and to prevent further entry of food.

ACUTE PULPITIS

A severe throbbing pain worsening with heat. Often very tender with pressure on the tooth. The cavity is cleaned and dressed with a quick-setting mixture, such as accelerated zinc oxide and eugenol, or one of the newer proprietary brands.

PERIAPICAL ABSCESS

Very severe pain unaffected by heat. Tooth is extremely tender to vertical pressure. Treatment is drainage, by extracting the tooth, or by making a hole in it with an aerotor bur. Pus can then drain out. Additional drainage may be obtained by incising any soft-tissue swelling with a scalpel blade. Hot salt water mouthbaths aid drainage by drawing pus from the root canal or extraction socket. Once excess pus has drained from the canal, the tooth is dressed with a root-canal antiseptic or antibiotic paste. When the canal is sterile it is then root filled.

PERIODONTAL ABSCESS

Tooth is usually tender to lateral pressure. It sometimes feels elongated, but is not affected by hot or cold. One removes the cause, such as a fish-bone, and cleans and syringes the area. If necessary, any swelling is incised to drain the pus. Hot saline mouth washes are used every two hours. In severe cases the tooth is extracted.

PERICORONITIS

The gum flap is syringed with warm salt water or hydrogen peroxide, and the patient may be given systemic antibiotics. The opposing tooth is sometimes extracted.

POSTOPERATIVE HAEMORRHAGE

Primary haemorrhage has been dealt with in Chapter XIII. However, the patient may return to the surgery with delayed or secondary haemorrhage.

He should be sat upright in the chair, and reassured. Under no circumstances should he rinse out his mouth. If much blood is present in the mouth it can be cleaned out with a damp gauze. This makes it easier to see the bleeding site and makes the patient feel better. The patient is asked to bite firmly on a clean damp gauze or handkerchief. If bleeding does not stop within 20 minutes the dentist must be consulted; if he is not available another dentist or a doctor should see the patient.

If bleeding does not stop with the above measures, the dentist may consider suturing the socket. The following should be sterilized and laid out in the surgery: local anaesthetic, suture thread and needles, needle holders, and scissors. A cellulose sponge or Russell's viper venom may be placed in the socket before suturing the mucosa.

If the haemorrhage is very severe the dentist might have to send the patient to hospital, so the number of hospital and ambulance station should always be on hand, next to the telephone.

DRY SOCKET

The patient comes back some 3 or 4 days after tooth extraction complaining of severe pain and bad taste. The socket is syringed with warm saline to remove any debris and is dressed, for example with iodoform, BIPP paste, or Whitehead's varnish on a ribbon of gauze. These have an anodyne effect, and prevent further packing of food into contact with the bare socket bone. The dressing is changed daily. Healing takes place from the base of the socket upwards.

QUESTIONS

1. A patient phones your surgery complaining of haemorrhage following extraction. What are the probable causes of this and what measures may be used to arrest the haemorrhage ? The dental surgeon is not immediately available.

2. What is the difference between a dental abscess and a periodontal (parodontal) abscess ? How is each treated ?

3. Discuss the cause and treatment of dry sockets.

4. Discuss the causes and treatment of toothache.

CHAPTER XV

PREVENTIVE DENTISTRY AND DENTAL HEALTH EDUCATION

PREVENTIVE DENTISTRY

THE study of aetiology (cause) and prevention of oral and dental diseases. Although usually referring to caries and periodontal lesions, it applies equally to malocclusion and fractured teeth.

Evidence of Aetiology

The causative factors of any disease are investigated by clinical, epidemiological, and experimental means.

1. CLINICAL

In searching for aetiological factors involved in the production of dental decay, clinical observations on the part of many dental surgeons led them to suspect the action of refined carbohydrates.

They noticed that many young children develop labial caries, which begins on the labial surfaces of the upper anterior deciduous teeth but later spreads to the other surfaces and teeth. It is usually associated with the prolonged use of comforter bottles or small feeders containing concentrated sugar solutions or fruit juices. Dummies dipped in honey produce a similar picture.

Another clinically observed phenomenon is that cervical caries is sometimes seen to occur suddenly in middle-aged men previously having little tooth decay. Quite frequently one finds that these patients have recently become fearful of the hazards of cigarette smoking, and have instead substituted continuous sweet sucking.

2. EPIDEMIOLOGICAL

This concerns the study of the prevalence of disease amongst different communities, ancient and modern. Old skulls show that in ancient times there was very little dental caries. Modern primitive peoples such as the Eskimoes and Maoris also had little decay until they made contact with civilization and its accompanying modern foods. Soon after they started to eat a 'civilized' diet, caries began to appear. Until then, Eskimoes had no word in their language for toothache.

Caries is more prevalent in countries enjoying the highest standards of living, with very high consumption of sugars. During the Second World War sugar consumption decreased in countries like Norway. This was soon followed by a corresponding fall in the caries rate. Soon after the war ended, caries again increased, indicating a direct relationship between sugar intake and caries prevalence.

Similar epidemiological studies have pointed to the relationship between poor oral hygiene and gingival inflammation.

3. EXPERIMENTAL

a. Human: In order to test the relationship between caries incidence and the intake of refined carbohydrates 400 people in Vipeholm, Sweden, were divided into 7 groups.

Group 1 (the control group) fed on a basic low-carbohydrate content diet, plus margarine to make up an adequate calorie intake.

Group 2 had basic diet plus sugar solution at mealtimes.

Group 3 had sweetened bread with meals.

Groups 4–7 had a basic diet plus sweets, toffees, caramels, or chocolates between meals.

RESULTS OF THE VIPEHOLM STUDY:

1. Less caries occurred when nothing sweet or sticky was taken between meals.

2. Large quantities of sugar in solution at mealtimes led to some increase.

3. Sugar in a sticky form at mealtimes led to a greater increase.

4. The greatest increase was with frequent consumption of sugar, in a sticky form, between meals.

5. Least decay occurred when no sugar was added to the basic diet.

6. In all cases the increase in caries was found to be halted and then reversed with withdrawal of refined carbohydrate from the diet.

b. Animal: Similar results have been obtained in rats. It has also been shown that caries only occurs in the presence of certain bacteria. These animals have also been used to demonstrate the effects of various foods on caries incidence, when taken during tooth formation. Refined carbohydrates do not induce caries when introduced direct to the stomach via a tube, thus indicating a local rather than a systemic effect.

DIETARY AND NUTRITIONAL CONTROL

In view of the relationship found between caries occurrence and the intake of refined carbohydrates, the latter must be strictly controlled. They should ideally be completely eliminated from the diet. If this is not possible such foods should only be taken at mealtimes, and never in a sticky form. Thus, chocolates cause less damage than do toffees. Sweet and sticky medicines should ideally be well diluted, taken through a straw direct to the back of the mouth after meals, and the mouth immediately rinsed with water. It has been suggested that fried foods coat the teeth and protect them from contact with refined carbohydrates. In addition they fill the stomach and lessen the demand for carbohydrate foods.

We have been concerned above with the elimination of local factors causing decay. However, a most important line of defence lies in improving the structure of teeth by ensuring that a balanced diet is taken during tooth formation. Thus, adequate intakes of calcium, phosphorus, fluoride, and vitamins A, C, and D are essential. Calcium and phosphorus are contained in milk, cheese, and liver, vitamins A and D in cod-liver oil, and vitamin C in fresh fruit and vegetables. Most of these are taken in adequate quantities by consuming normal, balanced meals. Only fluoride tends to be deficient, so other means of introducing this have had to be considered.

Fluoridation of the Public Water Supplies

In those areas where people drink water naturally containing up to one part of fluoride per million parts of water, there is much less decay than in regions without this protective factor. Scientists have discovered that by adding such an amount of fluoride to water deficient in this element, maximum benefit is obtained by the population, resulting in a substantial decrease in the incidence of caries.

Fluoride is perfectly safe, occurring naturally in many parts of the world in much higher concentrations than that recommended for caries prevention. Two and a half bathtubs full would have to be drunk before any toxic effects occurred.

Fluoride can be taken by the individual in tablets, salt, bread, or milk. However, all of these rely on the utmost co-operation on the part of parents and children to ensure adequate daily intake of fluoride during the years of tooth formation. With the best will in the world this is a difficult requirement to satisfy. However, fluoride in the water is safe, requires no individual effort, is considerably effective against decay, and is cheap and easy to insert automatically.

Topical Fluorides

Substantial reductions in caries incidence are obtained by applying fluorides to the surface of teeth after these have erupted into the oral cavity. The main means of applying fluorides are:—

1. Topical solutions.

2. Prophylactic pastes.
3. Toothpastes.
4. Mouthwashes.
5. Gels.
If used on patients drinking fluoridated water an additive effect is obtained.

TOPICAL SOLUTIONS

Sodium and stannous fluorides are used. An 8 per cent solution of stannous fluoride must be made up immediately prior to use or it will deteriorate and have no beneficial effect: 0·8 g. of stannous fluoride powder are added to 10 ml. of distilled water and the two are gently mixed together in a plastic container, plastic having no chemical effect on stannous fluoride.

After polishing the teeth, the solution is applied for 4 minutes, using cotton-wool wrapped around an orange-wood stick for all the accessible surfaces and unwaxed silk floss to take the solution between the teeth. The patient should not rinse his mouth for half an hour after the application.

Armamentarium:
Mirror, probe, tweezers.
Handpiece, rubber cup.
Saliva ejector.
Stannous fluoride powder.
Distilled water.
Cotton-wool rolls.
Orange-wood sticks.
Unwaxed silk floss.

PROPHYLACTIC PASTES

Special pastes used by dentists to polish patients' teeth. Some have fluoride incorporated into their substance whilst others have to be mixed at the chairside. They are applied to all surfaces of the teeth with a rubber cup and unwaxed silk floss. Immediately afterwards the patient is instructed to rinse his mouth to remove any residual paste, ensuring that none is swallowed.

TOOTHPASTES

Daily use of a fluoride toothpaste is advantageous in decreasing the rate of decay.

For maximum effect topical solution is applied yearly, prophylactic paste at each four-monthly recall visit, and fluoride toothpaste daily.

MOUTHWASHES

2 ml. of a 0·2 per cent solution of sodium fluoride are dispensed into a disposable plastic cup. The child takes the solution into his mouth, and swishes it backwards and forwards between the teeth for 2 minutes, before putting it back into the cup. Such a preventive measure may be carried out at the same time by a whole class of children.

GELS

Acidulated phosphate fluoride gels are inserted into special wax trays, which hold them in contact with the teeth for the requisite period of time.

MAINTENANCE OF ORAL HYGIENE

Oral hygiene: Sum of all the measures practised by dentist and patient to achieve a satisfactory state of oral cleanliness, and through this to attain and maintain maximum oral and dental health.
Oral cleanliness: State of the mouth as seen at examination.

Fibrous Foods

Meals should end with fibrous foods such as apples, carrots, nuts, or celery. These have a cleansing action by helping to remove food debris from the teeth. In addition they stimulate the periodontal tissues. Fibrous foods are also excellent substitutes for sweets and biscuits.

Bubble and Swallow

At the end of a meal water should be taken into the mouth, swished backwards and forwards between the teeth, and then swallowed. This assists the removal of food debris from between and around the teeth, and dilutes any acid products present in the oral cavity.

Muscular Action

Much cleansing of buccal and lingual surfaces is accomplished by the combined action of tongue, cheeks, and lips.

Toothbrushing

Teeth should be brushed immediately after each meal, especially after the last food of the day. The brush is laid against the gums and teeth with its bristles pointing rootwards (*Fig.* 43). The head of the brush is then rotated, pulling its bristles down along the gingivae and on to the teeth, in the direction of tooth eruption. The brushing technique should be used systematically, first in the maxilla and then in the mandible. One begins on the buccal aspects of the molars and then works round, via the anterior teeth, to the molars on the other side. The process is then repeated for the lingual surfaces. Finally the occlusal surfaces are scrubbed by moving the brush back and forth. Each area should be brushed at least ten times, ensuring maximum cleanliness of the teeth and maximum stimulation of the gingival tissues. For most purposes a medium or hard bristle or nylon brush may be used, but this is varied according to the patient's needs.

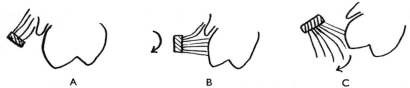

Fig. 43.—Brushing technique. A, Brush on gum; B, C, Bristles rotated on to tooth, clean dirt off tooth.

Toothpastes

Dentifrices can be obtained as pastes, powders, solid blocks, and liquids. These are supplementary to the brush, aiding the cleansing and polishing of *accessible* surfaces of the teeth. The main constituents are mild abrasives, soaps and detergents, colouring and flavouring agents. Additional substances such as ammonium salts, chlorophyll, penicillin, sodium N-lauryl sarcosinate, and fluorides have all been used, with varying degrees of success.

If a commercial paste is not available, salt and bicarbonate of soda are very cheap and effective substitutes.

Flossing

Silk floss is wrapped around two fingers and gently pulled backwards and forwards between the teeth, taking care to avoid damage to the gingivae.

The Dentist and Oral Hygiene

The dental surgeon's role is to ensure the complete elimination of decay and stagnation areas by scaling, polishing, and filling the teeth, providing dentures, and carrying out orthodontics as and when necessary. By these means he will ensure that no regions remain in the mouth whereby food can lodge and cause caries and gingivitis.

SUMMARY OF ORAL HYGIENE METHODS

1. BY PATIENT

Avoid sticky refined carbohydrates, especially between meals.
Eat cleansing, fibrous foods at the end of each meal.
Bubble and swallow.
Muscular activity.
Toothbrushing.
Flossing.
Regular visits to the dentist.

2. BY DENTIST

Elimination of decay and stagnation areas by scaling and polishing, conservation, prosthetics, orthodontics, and fissure sealants.
Advice on oral hygiene.

DENTAL HEALTH EDUCATION OF INDIVIDUALS AND THE COMMUNITY

Oral health, as well as general health, is only achieved by constant preventive measures as well as routine treatment. Education is carried out on two levels, for the individual and for the community. In this the good dental surgery assistant has an essential role to play. People often turn to her for advice, which she should be prepared and equipped to give.

Patients must be taught the causes of decay and gingivitis, being told especially of the parts played by refined carbohydrates, bacteria, and plaque. The latter can be demonstrated at the chairside with a disclosing solution or tablets. The patient's teeth are then polished, after which one can demonstrate that plaque is no longer present. The role of toothbrushing should be explained and the patient must be shown how to clean his teeth correctly. In addition, he should be told which foods to eat and which to avoid. Finally, he is instructed to visit the dentist at regular intervals.

The community as a whole may be taught to care for the mouth by means of group discussions, lectures, television, newspapers, and posters. Special importance must be attached to giving schoolchildren education in oral and dental health matters. It is at this stage that good habits can most easily be learnt, and bad ones discovered and discarded.

Many ancillary dental workers are now taking the examination leading to the Diploma in Dental Health Education awarded by the Royal Society of Health. Possession of this qualification will indicate to prospective employers that a high standard of knowledge and an ability to communicate have been demonstrated to the examiners.

QUESTIONS

1. What is the importance of scaling and polishing the teeth ? List the instruments and materials that you would prepare for this operation.

2. What are the results of lack of oral hygiene ? What measures for the care of the teeth and gums might be advocated for:—

   a. A woman of 30 with an upper partial acrylic denture ?

   b. A man of 60 wearing no denture with much of his natural dentition intact ?

3. What steps can a mother take to protect the dental health of her child ?

4. Discuss the arguments for and against fluoridation.

CHAPTER XVI

LOCAL AND GENERAL ANAESTHESIA AND ANAESTHETIC EMERGENCIES

General Anaesthesia: Loss of sensation produced by putting the patient to sleep, thereby preventing reception of pain stimuli by the brain.

Local Anaesthesia: A localized state of insensibility to pain produced by preventing conduction of stimuli along a nerve, by placing a chemical somewhere along its length.

Topical Anaesthesia: Loss of pain by application of anaesthetic sprays, solutions, pastes, and ointments to the surface mucosa or skin, from where they penetrate through the outer epithelium to reach the nerve-fibres.

INDICATIONS FOR GENERAL ANAESTHESIA

1. Acute infection at the usual site of injection, as the needle would carry bacteria to the deeper tissues. Also, local anaesthetics tend not to function in such areas.

2. Where the mouth cannot be opened sufficiently wide, for example with muscular spasm and temporomandibular joint disturbances.

3. Extra-oral drainage of facial and neck swellings.

4. Where there is a history of allergy to injection solutions.

5. Extraction of many teeth from all parts of the mouth.

6. Extraction or drainage of acutely abscessed teeth.

7. Major oral surgery including treatment of jaw fractures.

8. Full mouth conservation for severely mentally and physically handicapped patients, and the very nervous.

INDICATIONS FOR LOCAL ANAESTHESIA

1. Painful cavity preparation.

2. Extirpation of pulp.

3. Pulpotomy.

4. Extraction of teeth, especially where one cannot obtain the services of a separate anaesthetist, where the patient wishes to immediately drive a car, or where his medical condition precludes a

general anaesthetic (including disorders of the cardiac and respiratory systems).

5. Minor oral surgery, including apicectomy, gingivectomy, removal of cysts, drainage of abscesses by local incision.

6. Incorporation into dressings for painful sockets, ulcers, and wounds.

USE OF TOPICAL ANAESTHETICS

1. Prevention of pain from needles during injections.
2. Relief of painful sockets, ulcers, and wounds.
3. Reduction of sensitivity of oral mucosa for patients who retch during the taking of impressions or radiographs.
4. Prevention of gingival discomfort whilst taking copper ring impressions.

INJECTION APPARATUS

Syringes should be easily cleaned and sterilized. They mostly take anaesthetic solutions pre-packed in cartridges. These are slipped into the syringe and pierced by the reverse end of the needle which has previously been placed in position.

Needles

Obtained in a variety of lengths and diameters. It is easier to penetrate the tissues with thinner needles, but these are more readily broken. They are sometimes tapered, the tip being finely pointed, but that part nearest to the syringe being thicker for added strength. Long needles with short hubs are used in situations where the tip has to travel through a great deal of tissue, in an inferior dental block, for example. In other cases, maximum protection is afforded by short needles used with a long hub.

The same needle must never be used for more than one patient, as there is a risk of passing on the virus causing serum hepatitis. Nowadays it is common to use needles pre-sterilized in the factory by exposure to gamma rays.

PROPERTIES OF AN IDEAL ANAESTHETIC COMPOUND

1. Non-toxic.
2. Non-irritant.
3. Capable of being sterilized.
4. Rapid in onset.
5. Duration of anaesthesia sufficient for operation.

6. Anaesthetic effect temporary only, ideally wearing off immediately ae operation ends.

7. Must be capable of staying localized in the desired area.

Examples of local anaesthetics are cocaine (seldom used now), procaine, and lignocaine, which are described in Chapter XX.

Adrenaline, a vasoconstrictor, is sometimes added to cause localized constriction of the blood-vessels, preventing rapid loss of anaesthetic from the site. It therefore prolongs the period of action of the anaesthetic. Adrenaline is not normally used in patients with heart disease.

TYPES OF INJECTIONS

1. Regional blocks: inferior dental, mental, infra-orbital, posterior superior dental, greater palatine, sphenopalatine.
2. Infiltration.
3. Papillary.
4. Intra-osseous.

Inferior Dental Blocks

The needle is inserted into the tissues behind and above the last lower molar tooth. This causes anaesthesia of the inferior dental and lingual nerves, owing to their close proximity. Anaesthesia of the inferior dental nerve results in loss of sensation of all the lower teeth, and is therefore suitable for cavity preparation. However, for extractions, a supplementary buccal injection is also given. As the lip is also anaesthetized, patients must be warned to beware of biting it.

Infra-orbital and Mental Blocks

In these cases the needle is inserted into the mucosal reflection close to the corresponding foramen.

Posterior Superior Dental Blocks

Here the solution is injected distal to the maxillary tuberosity.

Greater and Sphenopalatine Blocks

As the palatal mucosa in these regions is firmly bound down to bone, these injections are given very slowly to prevent pain from excessive pressure on nerve-endings.

Infiltrations

Injection is made at the buccal reflection of mucosa overlying the root apex or site of operation.

Papillary

The needle is inserted directly into the interdental papilla.

Intra-osseous

When difficulty occurs in anaesthetizing a tooth for cavity preparation, a hole may be drilled through the bone itself, and anaesthetic solution actually placed into the hole. This is rarely used.

COMPLICATIONS FOLLOWING INJECTIONS

1. Fainting.
2. Failure of anaesthetic: due to faulty technique, old stock of solution, or anatomical variation.
3. Swelling: caused by oedema fluid, allergic response, or injection into a vein.
4. Broken needle: immediately hand the dentist a pair of artery forceps to grip that part of the needle remaining in the tissues.
5. Needle infection: to prevent organisms from being carried into the tissues, the mucosal surface is swabbed with antiseptic prior to injections with a sterile needle.
6. Pain: decreased by using sharp needles, and injecting slowly.

INHALATION ANAESTHESIA

A means of introducing a gaseous anaesthetic through the nose or mouth, via a mask or tube. The commonest inhalation anaesthetic agents are nitrous oxide, oxygen, and Fluothane (halothane).

Nitrous Oxide

First prepared in 1772. In 1798 Humphrey Davy inhaled it and found that his wisdom-tooth pain stopped. Early in the nineteenth century public demonstrations were given of the strange effects of this 'laughing gas'. In 1844 Horace Wells had a tooth taken out whilst under the influence of this gas, thus beginning the era of inhalation anaesthesia.

Oxygen is delivered from a black cylinder with a white collar, and nitrous oxide from a blue one. Fluothane or Trilene (trichloroethylene) is added from a small bottle incorporated in the circuit. The nose- or face-mask is held above or on the patient's nose and he is allowed to inhale the mixture. The anaesthetist controls the quantities of each gas reaching the patient, thus making the 'sleep' deeper or lighter, thereby controlling the patient's responses. The anaesthetic is deepened until the patient experiences no pain.

INTRAVENOUS ANAESTHESIA

A method whereby the anaesthetic is introduced to the body via a needle inserted into a vein, such as one on the inner aspect of the arm or on the back of the hand.

The skin is swabbed with a disinfectant and the needle is pushed through the skin into an underlying vein. The syringe plunger is slightly withdrawn to aspirate blood, thus ensuring that the needle is actually in the vein. A measured quantity of anaesthetic is then injected.

Indications for Intravenous Anaesthesia

1. Induction of anaesthesia: It is therefore unnecessary to apply a face-mask to conscious, nervous patients. As soon as they go to sleep from the effects of a single dose of intravenous drug, the anaesthetic is continued with gas.

2. Simple extraction of one or two teeth.

3. Conservation under general anaesthesia: occasionally patients are kept asleep by means of a continuous drip of drug into a vein. This is thought by some operators to be suitable for highly nervous patients. The dose is sometimes adjusted so that the patient is relaxed but virtually awake.

The most commonly used drug is methohexitone sodium (Brietal). Others are thiopentone and Epontol (propanidid).

PREPARATION OF PATIENT FOR ANAESTHESIA

The surgery assistant must ensure that the patient has not eaten during the four hours prior to anaesthesia, as there is a danger that this could cause vomiting, with the risk of vomit being inhaled and choking the patient. He should go to the lavatory as relaxation of his muscles might allow his bladder to empty during the anaesthetic. Dentures must be removed, and all tight clothing loosened. Written consent should be obtained for anaesthetic and operation.

The patient should be seated with his hips well back in the chair. It is useful first to remove the foot-rest of the chair, if there is one, to prevent patients bracing themselves against this during anaesthesia. Hands should either be placed in pockets or across the lap. Restraining straps are occasionally placed across the pelvis to stop the patient hurting himself whilst asleep.

THE OPERATION

A prop is placed between the teeth to keep the mouth open. As soon as the patient is asleep a gauze pack is carefully placed to separate the pharynx from the oral cavity, thus ensuring that no blood or debris is inhaled. A piece of cord attached to the pack prevents this being inhaled. If the operator wishes to change sides during the operation, a mouth-gag is applied to the side already operated on and slightly opened, allowing the original prop to be removed. It is essential to ensure that no blood is allowed to run backwards, and to ensure that the operator can see properly. The assistant should therefore continually be on hand with an efficient aspirator.

STAGES OF ANAESTHESIA

1. Induction.
2. Maintenance at stage of surgical anaesthesia.
3. Recovery.

SIGNS OF ANAESTHESIA

Patient breathes quietly and regularly.
The muscles are relaxed.
The pupils of the eyes get smaller.
The skin is usually pink with a slight bluish tinge as opposed to blackish colour due to anoxia or lack of oxygen.

POSTOPERATIVE CARE

All props and gags must be removed from the mouth, and the patient's head held gently forward to prevent blood or debris reaching the pharynx. It is essential to watch for vomiting or fainting. In the latter case, the patient's head is lowered and the anaesthetist informed immediately. Under no circumstances should the patient be left alone until he has fully recovered consciousness. He should not leave the building until in full possession of his faculties, and preferably accompanied by a responsible adult. Under no circumstances should he be allowed to drive a car for the rest of the day.

CARE OF ANAESTHETIC EQUIPMENT

It is essential to check anaesthetic equipment prior to each session, to ensure that everything is working correctly and safely. Otherwise a patient may come to harm. Gas machines should be checked by a skilled mechanic every six months. Anaesthetic emergency kits should be kept up to date, and should be on hand during the operation. Drugs with a limited shelf life must be checked to ensure that none have deteriorated.

ANAESTHETIC EMERGENCIES

Everyone is likely to be faced with a sudden emergency at some time during their life, be it in the surgery, at home, or in the street. The most important thing is to recognize what is wrong, and to know what to do. Putting this knowledge to prompt use may save a life, which justifies very careful study of this subject.

In the surgery there should be a fixed routine. Dentist, anaesthetist, and chairside assistant should know the part which each must play. The last named should immediately make available any emergency kit, sucker, and oxygen. A doctor or ambulance may be required, so the numbers of these should be kept next to the telephone.

Fainting (Syncope)

If the patient feels faint, or appears about to do so (i.e., looks pale, uneasy, and sweating), his head should be lowered between his knees or the chair should be tipped back so that his feet are up in the air and his head is below the level of his heart. This aids circulation of blood and thus oxygen to the brain. Sometimes spirits of ammonia are held below the nose to speed recovery. If the faint was caused by fear the patient should be reassured as he comes round. A drink of glucose may be given. It sometimes helps to prevent a feeling of faintness if the patient has a good meal before coming to the surgery for a local anaesthetic.

Epileptic Fit

The patient may suddenly lose consciousness. Occasionally he receives a warning sensation. During such an attack he may go rigid or undergo phases of alternate muscular contraction and relaxation. A gag must be placed between the teeth to prevent him biting his tongue. A napkin wrapped around a spoon forms a suitable gag. In addition the head is kept low to ensure blood-flow to the brain. Apart from these first aid measures, the patient is allowed to recover spontaneously.

Poisoning

The best treatment is to make the person vomit by placing two fingers at the back of his throat. Then he should be quickly sent to the nearest hospital. The poison should be sent with him to allow the doctor to identify it, and thus administer any neutralizing antidote. He may wash out the patient's stomach contents.

Respiratory Obstruction

The airway can become blocked by inhaled blood, mucus, tooth fragments, or vomit during operations under general anaesthesia. The anaesthetic is immediately stopped. Whilst the anaesthetist removes the pack and clears the airway, the attendant should stand by with sucker and emergency kit. It is often sufficient to give three or four sharp slaps between the shoulder-blades to dislodge the object. However, if it cannot be removed, a hole is made into the trachea (tracheotomy), so that air can pass straight to the lungs in spite of the blockage.

Respiratory Arrest

If breathing stops, air must be mechanically forced into the lungs. Delay can be fatal. This can be done with oxygen from an anaesthetic machine, or by mouth-to-mouth breathing.

MOUTH-TO-MOUTH BREATHING

An artificial method of filling the lungs with air. The patient is laid on his back and dentures are removed to avoid choking. The operator stands or kneels at the patient's side. The patient's head is extended well back and his lower jaw is held well forward, taking the tongue with it, thus ensuring that the airway remains open. Sometimes this alone allows breathing to begin. If not, take a deep breath and blow into the patient's mouth either directly or via a special airway. Pinch his nostrils shut to ensure that no air escapes from there. Blow until his chest rises, and then remove your mouth, allowing air to escape from his lungs. In the case of a child, your mouth should go over his mouth and nose. Inflation is continued at a rate of ten times a minute, until the patient starts to breathe on his own.

Whilst this is going on a second person sends for an ambulance.

Cardiac Failure

Stoppage of the heart means that even if air is taken into the lungs, it will not circulate to the brain. When deprived of oxygen the brain cells soon suffer irreversible damage. Presence, or absence, of a pulse may be detected at the wrist, temple, or neck. During cardiac arrest the pupils of the eyes are very dilated (large). The heart must be restarted immediately by external cardiac massage.

EXTERNAL CARDIAC MASSAGE

The patient is laid on his back, on a firm surface. The heel of one hand is placed in the centre of the chest, over the lower half of the sternum (breast bone), and the other hand is placed on top. Your full weight is then brought down with a sharp, firm movement, on to the sternum. This is depressed by $1\frac{1}{2}$ inches, compressing the heart which lies below. Blood is forced out of the heart into the circulatory system. Pressure is then relaxed, the chest expands, and the heart fills with blood. Excessive pressure could break the ribs. This process is repeated 60 times a minute (once a second), until the heart beats on its own. This may not be for several hours.

If necessary, cardiac massage and mouth-to-mouth breathing must be continued by the same person, doing first one for 20 seconds and then the other.

Cardiac Angina

The patient experiences sudden pain in the region of the sternum and left arm, brought on by effort. He should be instructed to remain perfectly still until the attack wears off. It may be helpful to crush a capsule of amyl nitrate under his nose. A doctor should be consulted.

Coronary Thrombosis

There is sudden pain in the stomach region, cyanosis (blue tinge of the skin), and a fall in the blood-pressure. Attacks are not necessarily brought on by exertion. Patients should be rested and given oxygen until a doctor arrives, or an ambulance takes them to hospital.

A SUITABLE EMERGENCY KIT

List with addresses and phone numbers of local doctors and hospitals.

Oxygen cylinders.
Aspirator.
Selection of anaesthetic airways.
Re-breathing bag.
Intubation tubes.
Adult- and child-size anaesthetic face-pieces.
Laryngoscope.
Tongue forceps.
Aromatic ammonia.
Amyl nitrate capsules.
Glucose.
Sterile syringes and needles.
Other drugs as suggested by the dentist or anaesthetist.
These must be continually checked and kept in perfect order.

QUESTIONS

1. What are the duties of the dental nurse during extractions under

general anaesthesia ? What are the risks associated with this type of anaesthesia ?

2. Describe how anaesthesia is produced when nitrous oxide and oxygen is administered to a patient for the extraction of a tooth. What preparations are required and what help would you give to the patient and dentist before, during, and after the procedure ?

3. For what reasons is a patient likely to faint in the dental surgery ? Describe the general principles of treatment.

4. Discuss the need for mouth-to-mouth resuscitation. How is it carried out?

CHAPTER XVII

RADIOGRAPHY

X-RAYS were first discovered in 1895 by Röntgen. They are produced when cathode rays strike a tungsten target within a sealed glass tube from which all air has been evacuated (*Fig.* 44). X-rays pass through soft tissues to produce a black image on a sensitized film. Calcified

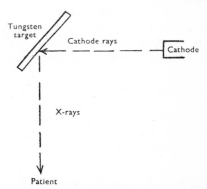

Fig. 44.—Cathode rays from a cathode hit a tungsten target, causing it to give off X-rays.

structures such as bones and teeth prevent their passage, causing a white or grey image on a black background. The resulting film is termed a 'radiograph'. In order to ensure maximum diagnostic value it is necessary to use the correct type of film for the purpose required. It must be carefully exposed and processed according to the instructions given by the manufacturer.

Radiographers are specially trained to take and process radiographs, whereas radiologists both take and interpret them. Dental radiographs are used to interpret and diagnose structures not seen at normal clinical examination.

Dental surgery assistants take or assist the dental surgeon in taking radiographs and in processing them. They must be able to mount a set of films correctly.

RADIATION HAZARDS IN THE DENTAL SURGERY

Care must be taken whilst using X-rays so as to ensure absolute safety for both patient and staff. Excessive radiation can damage tissues and organs, causing conditions such as necrosis of bone, tumours, and leukaemia. Thus the beam of X-rays is only directed on to the part necessary for diagnosis. In dentistry the rays are scattered around the area of the face and head. There is a danger of patients' genital organs being irradiated by reflected indirect rays, with a risk of damage to the reproductive cells. The chairside assistant can be subjected to both direct and indirect rays. She must *never* hold a film in patient's mouths, nor stand too close during exposure.

Protection for Patient and Operator

Patients should be subjected to as small a dosage of X-rays as is possible. Surgery assistants must therefore take great care in taking and processing films to avoid any repeats. The use of *fast* films enables exposures to be reduced. Apparatus should be frequently checked by an expert to ensure that no stray rays are emitted, and to detect any electrical faults.

X-ray beams may be reduced in width by a diaphragm at the exit aperture of the tube. This alters the size of the hole so that only the part under examination is irradiated. The tube-to-film distance controls the intensity of radiation reaching the film. As the distance increases the beam of X-rays is spread over a larger area, and the amount of radiation reaching the actual area under examination is reduced. Conversely, decreasing this distance increases the amount of radiation. Careful positioning of the tube decreases the rays reaching the gonads (reproductive organs). In addition the patient should wear a lead apron, which prevents the passage of X-rays. *This is especially important for young children and pregnant women.* Unless absolutely unavoidable the latter should never be exposed to radiation, as scatter rays could damage the foetus.

Whenever possible an X-ray-absorbing screen of lead should lie between operator and source of radiation. If many radiographs are taken a lead wall partition should be used. A viewing window is incorporated so that the operator can stand on the other side of the wall to view the patient whilst operating the machine. Alternatively, the operator can wear a lead apron over the front of the body to protect genital and other organs.

X-RAY FILMS

These consist of a transparent cellulose acetate or polythene base coated with silver bromide salts suspended in gelatin. They must be kept in a cool dry place, away from X-rays and any contaminating chemical fumes. Lead-lined boxes are the most suitable containers.

Developing Solution: Converts the exposed silver salts to a black silver deposit.

Fixer Solution: Dissolves off the unexposed silver and makes the image on the film permanent.

In order to ensure a consistently high standard it is important to follow carefully the manufacturers' *time and temperature* instructions.

DENTAL RADIOGRAPHS

These are divided into two main groups according to whether or not the film is placed within or outside the mouth during exposure. The actual view taken depends upon the purpose for which it is required.

1. Intra-oral

For examination of localized regions:—
a. Periapical.
b. Interproximal or bite-wing.
c. Occlusal.

2. Extra-oral

For examination of larger areas of the jaws, temporomandibular joints, and facial profile:—
a. True lateral.
b. Lateral obliques.
c. Postero-anterior.

Extra-oral films are often placed between intensifying screens in a cassette, which allows reduction of exposure time.

INTRA-ORAL EXAMINATION

Periapical

For a clear picture of the whole tooth plus the surrounding tissues. It is used to assess the state of health of pulp, dentine, cementum, periodontal membrane, and alveolar bone. This view is of great value during root-canal therapy.

A full-mouth periapical examination consists of fourteen films, seven for each jaw; one for each incisal, canine, premolar, and molar region.

The film is placed in the mouth against the palatal surface of the tooth to be examined, with the raised dot *towards* the tooth and tube. The tube is placed so that the X-rays pass at right-angles to the bisecting line between the long axes of tooth and film (*Fig.* 45).

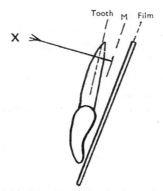

Fig. 45.—For accurate periapical radiographs the X-ray beam must come in at right-angles to the line (M) which divides the angle between film and tooth into two equal parts.

Bite-wings

For the detection of interproximal caries, and the pathology of the nearby bone.

The film is positioned with a special holder which is clenched between the teeth. The rays are directed between the teeth (*Fig.* 46).

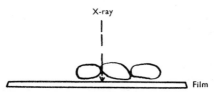

Fig. 46.—For bite-wing pictures the X-rays pass between the teeth and hit the film at right angles.

Occlusal

To investigate large areas of the maxilla or mandible for the presence of fractures, pathology, or unerupted teeth.

A large film is placed horizontally between the occlusal surfaces of upper and lower teeth. The rays are directed from above or below according to whether examination of mandible or maxilla is required.

EXTRA-ORAL EXAMINATION

True Lateral

To record the relationship between the teeth of upper and lower jaws, especially in orthodontics and prosthetics.

The film is held flat against the side of the head, and the rays are directed at right-angles to the film.

Lateral Obliques

These give a very clear picture of the mandible showing the state of the jaw-bone, as well as presence and position of erupted and unerupted teeth. There is, however, a less clear view of the maxillary tissues.

The position of patient, film, and tube are varied according to the view required. The film is placed against the outer aspect of the cheek, in contact with the part to be examined. The rays are projected from below, through the inner aspect of the mandible.

Postero-anterior

These films are valuable aids for detecting fractures of the skull and maxillary antral pathology. They give a general view of both sides of the maxilla and mandible plus the surrounding bone.

The film is held flat against the patient's forehead, nose, or chin. The rays are directed from behind the head to reach the film at right-angles to its surface.

PROCESSING

This is carried out in a darkroom or a specially constructed developing machine which can be used in the surgery. Darkroom illumination is by the use of a special safelight, usually orange in colour.

Developer and fixer must be checked to ensure that they are still usable. The former lasts for up to six weeks in the average surgery. The temperature of developing and fixing solutions are adjusted to that specified by the manufacturers.

The film is taken out of its packet and attached with the patient's name to the bottom of a hanger. Any paper insert is removed or it will interfere with processing. The lead backing should be retained. When sufficient has accumulated it should be sold or sent to a charitable organization. The film is immersed in developer for the correct length of time for that temperature, slightly agitating the hanger to dislodge any air-bubbles from the film. It is then rinsed in running water for 15 seconds to remove any remaining developer, after which it is placed in fixer for 15 minutes. It should not be examined in white light until all the ' creamy colour ' has disappeared. At this stage the film is transferred to running water and washed for 15 minutes. It is then hung in a dust-free atmosphere to dry. At *no time* during processing should any finger marks be allowed to get on to the film as they can mask the diagnosis.

FILING

When dry, films are usually mounted on a plastic sheet with the dot facing *away* from the plastic (i.e., towards the observer). The date, name, and case number *must* be written on the mount. Films are then placed in envelopes and stored either with the patient's record cards or in an index. They can be a most important source of information regarding a person's identity and are usually stored and kept for several years because of this.

FAULT FINDING IN RADIOGRAPHY

It is of the utmost importance to understand the reasons for poor radiography. The following list shows common faults and suggests ways in which they may be avoided.

Faint Image

The picture details cannot be properly seen.

a. This can be due to insufficient exposure because of a faulty time switch or a good one that is not fully depressed throughout the period of exposure. Also the X-ray cone may have been too far away from the face (it should be just off the skin surface).

b. Another cause may be incomplete development due to too short a time in the developer, too low a temperature, or worn-out developer.

Partial Image

Only part of the film bears an image.

a. Some of the film might not have been exposed to the X-rays due to incorrect positioning of the machine. The central rays should be aimed to pass through the centre of the film.

b. Part of the film will not be reached by developer if it contacts another film or the side of the tank during development, or if some of the wrapper still adheres to the film.

Fog

A generalized grey appearance over the whole film makes picture interpretation very difficult.

a. Accidental exposure to light.

b. Wrong safelamp filter, too bright a bulb, bulb too near bench top (should be about 4 feet away).

c. Chemical contamination.

d. Scattered radiation from a nearby X-ray machine (therefore store film in lead-lined box).

e. Storage of film in a warm room.

f. Old film stock.

g. Excessive development time, or too high a developing temperature.

White Marks

Grey or white spots are sometimes seen on radiographs.

a. Air-bubbles may be caught against the film when it is placed in the developing tank. The hanger should therefore be agitated a few times to dislodge them, as bubbles prevent developer reaching the emulsion with resultant lack of an image at that spot.

b. Similar blotches occur if fixing solution is splashed on to the film prior to development.

Herringbone Pattern

This pattern is embossed on to the metal foil backing. If the film is used with its backing facing the tube the pattern is reproduced on the picture. It is, therefore, important to ensure that the *raised dot faces the tube.*

Mottling

a. A generalized mottling may appear if the film is subject to too high a temperature.

b. Also if grossly differing temperatures are used in developing, fixing, and washing baths.

Dense Image

If the picture is very dark it is not possible to see the points for diagnosis.

a. Over-exposure.

b. Developer too warm.

c. Prolonged development time.

d. Light reaching the film by using the wrong darkroom filter or by not having a light-tight darkroom.

Blurred Image

Due to movement of the film, patient, or tube.

QUESTIONS

1. What are the hazards of excessive radiation and how may any danger to yourself and the patient be minimized ?

2. What are the reasons for taking radiographs in dentistry?
Describe the method of taking:—

a. An intra-oral film to show the apical conditions of an upper
central incisor.

b. Bite-wing films to show the interstitial caries in premolar and
molar teeth.

3. What errors can occur in the taking and processing of intra-oral
X-ray films? Describe the effect of any one which you have mentioned.

4. Describe the contents of an X-ray film packet. How would you
process the film?

CHAPTER XVIII

CHILD DENTAL HEALTH INCLUDING ORTHODONTICS

AIMS OF CHILDREN'S DENTISTRY (PAEDODONTICS)

1. Education of parent and child in the importance of oral health and in the prevention of dental disease.
2. Prevention of unnecessary pain, sepsis, extractions, and general anaesthetics.
3. Prevention of damage to underlying permanent successors by abscesses or extraction of deciduous teeth.
4. To accustom children to dentistry before fears develop.
5. Prevention of orthodontic anomalies due to early loss of deciduous teeth.
6. Early detection of other dental anomalies.
7. Avoidance of stagnation areas by means of orthodontic therapy, conservation, and prosthetics.

PATIENT MANAGEMENT

The approach and manner used by dentists and staff: (a) To help the patient feel confident and happy in the dental surgery; (b) To attain and maintain maximum oral and dental health.

Those involved in patient management are children, their parents, dentists, dental surgery assistants, and receptionists.

THE CHILD

Patients may be quite happy in the surgery, or might be frightened and/or naughty. It is of the utmost importance to determine which of these apply, as different lines of approach are required in each case. A very full history is therefore essential. A good surgery assistant can be very helpful in this respect, as both the child and its mother will often speak more readily to her than to the dentist.

Introduction of the Child to Dental Procedures

It is sometimes a good idea to let the child come when a parent or older child is being treated, provided that the latter is a good and calm patient. Small children are often brought to the surgery for morning appointments, when they tend to be less tired and irritable.

It is useful to have a few books and comics in the waiting room. Toys should only be included if they are of the type that will not get the child over-excited and tired before seeing the dentist. Small children may claim a toy and wish to take it home. Allow them to do this, and ask them to bring it back next time. This provides a link with the surgery. The good surgery assistant can do so much to help young patients to feel at ease and confident. Always use the child's name. Talk to him or her about favourite books and television programmes and with older children about school and games. Very young children like having their clothes admired, or to be told how big or tall they are. All these techniques are means of making a satisfactory contact with young patients.

If possible the dental surgeon will first interview parent and child outside the surgery, perhaps in the office or waiting room. If the dentist is seated he looks less like a giant and is more on a level with the child. A full history is taken from the parent, including the child's social background, school, games, brothers and sisters, and previous dental care.

Difficult and Naughty Children

An abnormal reaction to a normal dental situation may not be connected with dentistry, especially in a child that is usually well behaved in the surgery. For example, starting school or the arrival of a new baby into the family often upsets children. In such cases dentistry simply provides an outlet for the child's feelings. In these cases kindness and tolerance for a few visits, with little actual treatment carried out, will often work wonders.

In the case of children making a noise and exhibiting other signs of a temper tantrum, the dentist will often exclude parents from the surgery, as the child is then less likely to make an exhibition of itself. With such a child the dentist will be firm but not forceful. If the child refuses to sit in the chair he may be picked up and firmly, but gently, placed in it. He is told exactly what is going to be done, for example, polishing of the teeth. At such a time it is essential for the dentist to have absolute control of the situation, so under no circumstances should the parent or surgery assistant interfere with this relationship.

Examination of the Child

If possible the child is allowed to climb into the dental chair unaided. The chair should then be adjusted so that the child's head, neck, and spine are in a straight line. Children often slide down, with buttocks forward and chin down on the chest, which makes it difficult to see into the mouth. Remember that for very young children dental equipment appears very frightening, so little should be on show. The dentist may be seated and the child standing with his face or back to him so that he no longer looks like a giant. It may be possible to examine the nervous child away from the dental surgery, perhaps in the waiting room. Very young children may be examined sitting on their mother's lap whilst she sits in the dental chair.

Babies are examined lying on their backs across their mother's knees, the child's head resting on the dentist's lap.

Conversation

This is best restricted to dentist and child, with parents and staff looking on but not interfering. Words such as 'pain', 'needle', and 'drill' should be avoided. Instead, a simple vocabulary is established, substituting everyday words in place of the dental ones. Examples are 'spoon' for the excavator or bur, 'buzzer' for the handpiece. For cavity-probing words such as 'feel' and 'count teeth' can be used. Sometimes during the drilling of teeth children become almost hysterical with laughter when the word 'tickle' has been used. A syringe can be a 'squirter to put your teeth to sleep'. Rubber cup, bristle brush, or bur can be replaced by 'my toothbrush'. The ingenious dental surgery assistant can be most helpful to her dental surgeon.

Introduction of the Child to Instrumentation

It is essential for everything to be explained so that the child is continually reassured. The dentist might start with a rubber cup in his hand, using it to polish first his own finger-nails, then the child's, finally using it to clean the child's teeth. Toothpaste may be used. After this performance the rubber cup is transferred to a handpiece held in the hand and the procedure repeated. Eventually the handpiece is attached to the engine arm, by which time the child should have some confidence in the dentist. Once the actual procedure commences the child can be allowed to control the situation by first telling the dentist when to 'stop and start', and later to signal his instructions by raising a hand. In this way the child is introduced to quick, simple, and painless procedures.

Later, brushes, burnishers, and other instruments are substituted for the rubber cup, and the child willingly accepts it all. Exactly how far to go on each occasion depends upon the child, his age, temperament, and intellect.

Fear on the Part of a Patient

Fear is divided into two types, according to the aetological factors involved.

a. OBJECTIVE

In this case apprehension is associated with an adverse previous experience such as painful fillings and injections, or a frightening general anaesthetic, especially after toothache and loss of sleep.

b. SUBJECTIVE

This is based on personal feelings and attitudes and not actual experiences. Stories of terror from parents and friends, and fear of the unknown are included in this group.

Early Visits to the Dentist

Many fears are prevented when children are brought to the dentist before their third birthday. Ideally they should visit him before their teeth erupt as:—

1. They become used to a surgery and its equipment at an early stage and are not scared by lights, the sound of drills, and instruments.

2. Early dietary advice and dental health education may be given to child and parent.

3. Little or no treatment is usually necessary at this stage.

4. When this is needed it will be minimal and painless.

5. It avoids the difficulty of treating a child who has already had toothache and extraction.

ENDODONTIC TREATMENT OF DECIDUOUS TEETH

Deciduous teeth require endodontic therapy when the pulp is involved by infection or trauma. The treatment plan depends upon whether or not the pulp is vital.

Treatment of Vital Pulps

Pulp capping, vital pulpotomy, and devitalization are all used on vital deciduous pulps. Pulp capping has already been described (Chapter XII). It is only used for very small, non-infected exposures, produced accidentally during cavity preparation, when the tooth is not painful, and when there is only minimal pulpal bleeding. Pulpotomy is the treatment of choice for all other vital pulps. However, if it is difficult to treat a child and he will not have a local anaesthetic, then a devitalization technique is used.

DEVITALIZATION AND MUMMIFICATION

The exposed vital pulp is covered with devitalizing paste, over which is placed a small piece of cotton-wool and then a quick-setting dressing. The patient is sent away for a week, being told to take an analgesic tablet if any pain is experienced that night. The paste kills off the pulp, and then preserves it in a mummified state.

The following week the dressing is removed and non-vital pulp remnants are cleared out from the coronal pulp chamber with sterile burs and excavators, the root canals not being touched. The cavity is lined with quick-setting zinc oxide and eugenol, and then filled with amalgam.

Armamentarium:

Mirror, probe, tweezers.
Plastic instruments.
Excavators.
Rubber dam, clamps, frame, forceps.
Handpiece and burs.
Devitalizing paste.
Cotton-wool rolls and pellets.
Quick-setting zinc oxide and eugenol.
A TYPICAL DEVITALIZING PASTE:
Paraformaldehyde.
Procaine.
Powdered asbestos.
Vaseline.
Carmine.

Vital Pulpotomy

The removal of the coronal portion of pulp; that part adjacent to the exposure and therefore infected.

The tooth is anaesthetized and isolated with a rubber dam. Any remaining caries is removed and the cavity is washed with saline. The roof of the pulp cavity is then cut away to expose the pulp, and the whole coronal pulp is removed with a sharp round bur or excavator. The pulp chamber is again washed with saline and dried with sterile cotton pellets. Only pulp in the root canals remain. Bleeding on their surface should stop in a few minutes.

A pellet moistened with formocresol is placed in contact with the pulp stump for 5 minutes. The liquid is very caustic, so care should be taken to keep it off the fingers. The pellet is removed and the chamber is dried with another pellet.

A thick paste of zinc oxide and equal parts of eugenol and formo-cresol is placed over the stumps. The cavity is then lined with oxy-phosphate cement and the tooth is then restored.

Treatment of Non-vital Pulps, including those associated with an Abscess

The coronal pulp chamber is opened with a bur and thoroughly cleaned of necrotic (dead) pulp debris. If the tooth is abscessed, pus is allowed to drain out at this stage. A small pledgelet of cotton-wool is dipped in a sterilizing agent such as beechwood creosote, and any excess. liquid is removed by laying the pledgelet on a cotton-wool roll. The pledgelet is placed on the floor of the chamber over the entrances to the root canals, and covered with a quick-setting dressing.

The dressing is changed weekly until the pulp chamber is sterile. Then the coronal chamber is thoroughly cleaned, washed, dried, lined with a quick-setting cement, and filled with amalgam (*Fig.* 47).

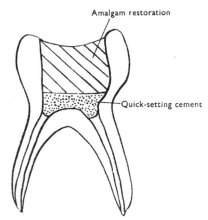

Amalgam restoration

Quick-setting cement

Fig. 47.—Filling of non-vital deciduous tooth.

TRAUMATIC INJURIES TO THE TEETH

Deciduous and permanent anterior teeth may be injured in the home, in the school playground, or on the sports field.

Types of Injury

1. Completely knocked out (avulsed).
2. Partially displaced (subluxed): buccally, lingually, incisally, or apically.

3. Loosened but remaining in place.
4. Immediate loss of vitality.
5. Concussed (unconscious): these may later recover or die.
6. Fractured.

Treatment of Knocked-out Teeth

These are sometimes replanted in the socket. In this case a splint is used to hold the tooth firmly in position until re-attachment takes place. The tooth is usually root filled before replacement.

If the tooth is left out, the dentist must decide whether to place a denture in the mouth at this time or to close the gap orthodontically.

Partially Displaced Teeth

These are often replaced into their original position and then splinted as above.

Loosened Teeth

A splint is usually cemented on to the teeth, and left for between 3 and 10 weeks depending upon the severity of the mobility.

SPLINTS

These are cemented on to loose teeth to hold them steady during eating, thus giving them adequate rest and a chance to recover fully.

An alginate impression is taken, often using a lower tray even for the upper teeth. A metal model is then constructed. From this the technician makes a splint of acrylic, silver, shellac or other thermoplastic material.

Non-vital Teeth

If left, the pulps of such teeth become necrotic and break down to form an abscess. They are therefore removed, and a root-canal filling is placed to occlude the pulp cavity.

However, before such a step is taken one must ensure that the pulp is really non-vital and not simply concussed (unconscious). The tooth is therefore kept under observation and pulp tested over a period of about 10 weeks before a decision is made.

Fractured Incisors

These are classified according to the tissues involved:—
Class 1: Enamel only.
Class 2: Enamel and dentine.
Class 3: Enamel, dentine, and pulp.
Class 4: Root.

ENAMEL FRACTURES

Rough edges are smoothed and polished with sandpaper disks and rubber cups.

FRACTURES OF ENAMEL AND DENTINE

In such cases the tooth may hurt when the patient eats hot and cold foods. Exposed dentine must therefore be protected by means of calcium hydroxide or zinc oxide and eugenol, covered by a cast silver cap or a stainless-steel preformed crown. The dressing is removed after 3 months, when a layer of secondary dentine has been deposited. At this stage the remaining tooth tissue is built up with a composite filling material, or a crown is constructed.

CROWNS

Modified three-quarter crowns may be used until the patient is about 16 years of age. With such crowns there is no danger of exposing the pulp, as only minimal preparation of the tooth is necessary. If normal crown preparation is attempted on a tooth with a large pulp, this would be immediately exposed.

Pulpal Exposures

Minute exposures of the pulp are covered with calcium hydroxide, over which is placed a zinc oxide dressing within a temporary crown as indicated above. This is left in place for about 4 months.

If the exposure is larger and the root apex is complete, the pulp is removed and replaced by a root canal filling. However, if there is an open apex a pulpotomy is performed. The living pulp remnants in the root then allow its completion.

PULPOTOMY

This is partial removal of the pulp, as opposed to pulpectomy, which is complete removal. Pulpotomy allows completion of the roots of young vital incisors. The coronal pulp is removed with a sharp excavator and the stump is covered with calcium hydroxide paste. Over this is placed a quick-setting zinc oxide and eugenol cement, and then an amalgam filling. After a time the open apex begins to close and the root elongates.

Injured Deciduous Teeth

If these have been displaced they may be left in the new position unless preventing closure of the mouth. In the latter case they are replaced in position, provided that in so doing the underlying developing permanent teeth are not damaged. Otherwise they are extracted.

SPACE MAINTAINERS

These are appliances used to replace teeth lost by caries or trauma, in order to prevent the teeth on either side of the remaining gap drifting towards each other. Some are fixed to the teeth whilst others are removable. Removable ones take the form of dentures, with or without teeth on the saddle area.

Fixed space maintainers are extended from the tooth in front, across the space, to contact the tooth behind. They are attached to one or both of the teeth next to the gap. Fixed space maintainers may consist of projections from gold inlays or stainless-steel bars welded to stainless-steel crowns or bands.

PRINCIPLES OF ORTHODONTIC THERAPY

Many children today have jaws which are too small to accommodate all their teeth. Others have minor irregularities, such as teeth which have erupted into the wrong position or are rotated. In yet another group, the jaws themselves are in an unsatisfactory relationship to each other. Most of these may be corrected by orthodontic therapy.

Malocclusion

A condition in which the cusps of upper and lower teeth do not meet in the normal way.

Orthodontics

The study of cause, prevention, and treatment of irregularities of shape of the jaws, and position of teeth. It is derived from the Greek words 'orthos' meaning straight, and 'odons', a tooth.

Aetiology of Malocclusion

1. Genetic, e.g., inheritance of small jaws from one parent and large teeth from the other.
2. Prolonged retention of deciduous teeth leading to displacement of the permanent successors.
3. Early loss of deciduous teeth.
4. Missing teeth.
5. Supernumerary or extra teeth, causing displacement of other teeth during eruption.

Orthodontic Treatment

By extraction of teeth, with or without the use of an orthodontic appliance.

Before treatment the dentist makes a full diagnosis and treatment plan. This involves careful examination of the patient, including the taking of radiographs, photographs, and study models.

ORTHODONTIC APPLIANCES
1. Fixed

Consist of wires attached to bands cemented on to the teeth, so that the patient cannot remove them from his mouth. This technique is time-consuming and is therefore limited to the treatment of more complex cases.

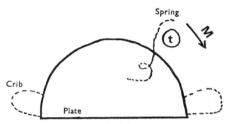

Fig. 48.—Diagram of a simple removable orthodontic appliance. The spring moves the tooth (t) in the direction of movement (M). Cribs aid retention of the plate.

2. Removable (*Fig.* 48)

Consist of wires and screws embedded in an acrylic plate which can be inserted in the mouth and taken out, by the patients. The springs are of differing shapes, lengths, and thicknesses, depending upon their function.

a. CRIBS

Wires gripping a tooth to help retain an appliance in the mouth.

b. LABIAL BOW

A long wire in front of the anterior teeth, which is used to aid retention of a plate and to retract several incisor teeth together.

c. SPRINGS

Used to move individual teeth. When pressure is applied to a tooth it tends to move away from the spring. Springs are placed mesially, distally, palatally, or buccally according to the desired direction of tooth movement. A combination of these is sometimes used for more complex movements, for example to rotate a tooth.

d. SCREWS

Normally used to move more than one tooth at a time. As the patient turns the screw himself, usually twice a week, less frequent visits to the dentist are needed.

EXTRACTIONS IN ORTHODONTICS

In patients with jaws small in comparison with the size of the teeth there is often insufficient room for all of these teeth to erupt into their correct position. It is therefore necessary to extract selected teeth to make more room. First premolars are commonly removed for this purpose, but other teeth may be extracted.

QUESTIONS

1. Discuss the part you can play in minimizing the distress of a young child on his first visit to the dentist.
2. Why do children require orthodontic treatment? Describe an upper removable appliance.
3. A child aged six comes to the surgery with a gumboil next to a deciduous molar tooth. How would the dentist treat it?
4. Discuss the treatment of fractured incisors in children.

CHAPTER XIX

SOME DISEASES OF CHILDHOOD

I<small>T</small> is important for all people who work with children, including dentists and their assistants, to know something of the common diseases of childhood. In this way one can recognize them early and prevent their spread to other patients and staff.

Table III.—A<small>CUTE</small> S<small>PECIFIC</small> F<small>EVERS</small>

D<small>ISEASE</small>	C<small>AUSATIVE</small> O<small>RGANISM</small>	I<small>NCUBATION</small> P<small>ERIOD</small> (days)	D<small>URATION</small> <small>OF</small> S<small>KIN</small> E<small>RUPTIONS</small> (days)	Q<small>UARANTINE</small> P<small>ERIOD</small> (days)	
				Patient	Contact
Measles	Virus	10–14	4	10	14
German measles	Virus	14–21	1–2	7	21
Chicken-pox	Virus	11–21	1–2	Until lesions heal	21
Mumps	Virus	14–28	—	7 days after swelling subsides	28
Whooping cough	Bacterium	2–14	—	21	14
Scarlet fever	Bacterium	1–3	2	7	7

Most of the diseases to be considered in this section fall under the heading of acute infective fevers, but rheumatic fever has also been included. The main manifestations of the acute fevers are summarized in *Table III.*

ACUTE SPECIFIC FEVERS

A number of infectious diseases all have one thing in common—a rise in temperature. Most are characterized by skin eruptions (exanthematous fevers). The causative organism may be a virus or a bacterium.

GENERAL METHODS OF TREATING ACUTE FEVERS

The patient should be put to bed in a warm, well ventilated room. A light nourishing diet consisting chiefly of fluids should be given. Drugs and tepid sponging are valuable in reducing the temperature. All the patient's utensils should be kept separate and carefully sterilized.

Measles

A virus infection spread by droplet spray during coughing and sneezing.

After incubation a respiratory inflammation begins: sneezing, running eyes and nose, and photophobia. This is the most infectious stage, so the patient should be isolated. On the second day of this catarrhal stage Koplik's spots may be seen on the buccal mucosa; they look like 'grains of salt' and disappear quickly. There is a rise in temperature of up to 103° F. and a hard type of cough. The face is puffy and swollen, especially around the eyes. The rash appears first around the face, near the hairline and behind the ears. Red spots group to form dusky red blotches. The rash spreads to the trunk and limbs, but fades within a few days. The temperature also falls during this period.

Rubella (German Measles)

A virus infection spread by direct contact and by droplet spray.

The onset is less acute than that of measles, and the patient is not so ill. General symptoms are headache, nasal catarrh, slight pyrexia, and malaise.

The rose-pink rash appears on the first day, beginning on the face, and spreading in crops over the trunk and limbs during the week. The rash can be seen under the skin before eruption, having a fine 'cobweb' appearance. The small lymphatic glands behind the ears harden and feel like 'gunshot', and the occipital lymph-glands are also affected.

This illness is generally a mild one. Complications are rare, unless it occurs during the first three months of pregnancy when the embryo is forming. The virus can penetrate the placenta which normally protects the growing foetus. The result can be disastrous, as the rapidly developing cells can be attacked, causing congenital deformity and heart disease. It is thus important for young girls to get German measles or be immunized against it before reaching childbearing age.

Chicken-pox

A virus infection known to be associated with the causative organism of shingles. Spread is by droplet infection, or by hands and clothing of contacts.

The onset is mild. The patient feels poorly, with a slight rise of temperature. The first sign may be the appearance of a rash. This starts on the trunk, especially on the back, and then spreads to face and limbs.

Red papules appear first, changing quickly to vesicles, and then to pustules. This is followed in a few days by scabs, which fall off. All types of the above lesions may be present at the same time in various parts of the body. Isolation continues until all 'crusts' have disappeared.

Mumps (Epidemic Parotitis)

A virus infection which spreads by droplet infection through the respiratory tract.

The patient complains of headache, sore throat, and a rise of temperature. This is followed by swelling of one or both parotid glands. The swelling thus appears behind the angle of the jaw. The overlying skin is tense and shiny. Eating and swallowing cause pain and the mouth may not open easily. The mouth is dry and the parotid duct opposite the upper molar teeth is reddened. The submandibular and submental glands may also enlarge. After about ten days swellings disappear and the temperature goes down.

Scarlet Fever

This is caused by the haemolytic streptococcus. It is mainly spread by droplet infection. Organisms enter a body via the throat. Children between 5 years and adolescence are the most vulnerable age-group.

The onset is sudden, with sore throat, headache, vomiting, and pains in back and limbs. The throat is very red and the tonsils covered with exudate (matter which passes out into tissue through vessel walls when inflammation is present). The tongue is heavily furred and looks like the surface of a strawberry (known as 'strawberry tongue'). The pulse rate is rapid and the temperature rises to about 103° F.

On the second day a rash appears on neck, shoulders, and chest, but not on the face. However, a white circle (circumoral pallor) develops around the nose and mouth. The body rash forms pink areas of scarlet spots which blanch on pressure. It fades in about a week and is followed by desquamation.

Whooping Cough (Pertussis)

A respiratory infection caused by the pertussis bacillus. One attack should confer immunity for life. It is spread by droplets during the coughing bouts, and is most virulent in the first two weeks before the ' whoop ' is heard. First there is a catarrhal stage, rather like a feverish cold, possibly preceded in the very young by bronchitis, and in older people by laryngitis.

When the disease is well under way coughing is followed by a long inspiratory 'whoop'. The patient appears to be reaching a point of asphyxia, and is greatly distressed. Coughing may be followed by vomiting. This stage lasts from 3 to 6 weeks.

Occasionally an ulcer appears below the tongue, as this repeatedly rubs against the incisor teeth during coughing.

Acute Rheumatic Fever

A condition caused by haemolytic streptococcus. Onset of the fever is preceded by a sore throat about 7 to 21 days beforehand. This is followed by a feeling of illness, high temperature, and much sweating.

Characteristic is pain in the joints and limbs, which become tender and swollen. Especially affected are knees, ankles, and wrists. The pain moves about from limb to limb.

The heart may be severely affected by acute rheumatic fever. Any further infection reaching the heart may cause the very serious disease bacterial endocarditis. Therefore, before dental treatment such as extractions and scaling patients are normally treated with a prophylactic dose of penicillin. Some children have such an antibiotic daily.

QUESTIONS

1. Write brief notes on:—
a. Carrier.
b. Incubation.
c. Virus infection.
d. Vesicle.
2. Discuss the general signs, symptoms, and treatment of acute fevers.
3. What is rheumatic fever ? Of what significance is it to dental surgeons ?
4. Compare and contrast Measles and German Measles.

CHAPTER XX

DRUGS AND DENTAL PRACTICE

IT is not only interesting but essential for all connected with dentistry to know something about the drugs used in dental practice.

LIST OF DRUGS

Absorbable gelatin sponge: A haemostatic agent used in bleeding sockets and cyst cavities. As it is resorbed in six weeks there is no need for the dentist to remove it.

Aconite and iodine: A disclosing solution to detect plaque on tooth surfaces.

Adrenaline: A vasoconstrictor applied to bleeding points in order to stop haemorrhage. It is also incorporated into local anaesthetics in order to localize the area of action.

Alcohols: Mixtures of varying concentrations of ethyl alcohol in water. Methylated spirit is 95 per cent alcohol and 5 per cent wood naphtha. A 70–95 per cent solution is antiseptic on mucosa, so is used prior to injections. It is astringent at more than 65 per cent and rubefacient at more than 50 per cent. Very dilute solutions act as refrigerants. With rapid evaporation they make the skin feel cool, e.g., eau de cologne used to cool fevered brows. Applied locally, alcohol is an obtundent; hence the application of whisky next to an aching tooth.

Alum: A styptic and astringent.

Ammonia: Acts as a stimulant when held under the nose of a fainting patient.

Aniline dyes: Powerful antiseptics, e.g., proflavine, gentian violet.

Aspirin and its compounds (Aspirin, caffeine, paracetamol): An antipyretic.

Barbiturates: A group of synthetic chemicals derived from barbituric acid. According to the actual drug and dose one may alter the length of action to obtain sedation (long-acting groups), hypnosis (medium- and short-acting), anaesthesia (short-acting), and premedication (short-acting).

Beechwood creosote: A root-canal antiseptic. It is very caustic. Any splashing on to the skin should be well neutralized with glycerin, and the remnants washed away with running water.

Benzocaine: Used in local anaesthetic lozenges prior to taking impressions of patients with sensitive palates. Also before eating with a very sore throat.

BIPP paste: Bismuth, iodoform, and paraffin paste used to fill apicectomy cavities and septic sockets.

Brietal: An intravenous anaesthetic.

Calcium hydroxide: A white powder soluble in water. For capping exposed pulps and sub-lining very deep cavities, where it stimulates the formation of secondary dentine, e.g., calxyl.

Carbolized resin: An obtundent and antiseptic temporary filling. Also a haemostat and anodyne for the treatment of painful extraction sockets.

Cetrimide (Cetavlon, Savlon): Antiseptic and detergent. Used as a 1 per cent solution (with the addition of 0·5 per cent sodium nitrate to prevent rusting) for sterilizing surgical instruments. The 1 per cent solution is also used to clear cyst cavities and extraction sockets of pus, mucus, and other debris. A 1 per cent cream is used to pack dry sockets.

Chloral: A hypnotic.

Chloramine: An antiseptic solution used to irrigate wounds (1 per cent), to cleanse mucous membranes (0·1 per cent), and to irrigate root canals (5 per cent).

Chloroform: Clear colourless liquid. Used as a general anaesthetic. It acts as a solvent for wax and gutta percha, the latter forming chloropercha.

Chromic acid: Dark purple crystals, very soluble in water. A 10 per cent solution is used as an antiseptic in the treatment of pericoronitis. It is left on for about 30 seconds and the mucosa is then swabbed with neutralizing hydrogen peroxide.

Clove Oil: A common dental anodyne.

Cocaine: One of the first local anaesthetics. Seldom used now.

Codeine: An analgesic.

Creosote: Bactericide used to sterilize root canals.

Dakin's solution: *See* Sodium hypochlorite.

Easlick's paste: Paraformaldehyde devitalizing paste used to treat infected deciduous pulps.

Ephedrine nasal drops: For relief of nasal congestion and sinusitis.

Ethyl chloride: A colourless liquid used for general and local anaesthesia. It is sprayed on to a mucosal abscess prior to incision and drainage. It also provides a cold stimulus for testing pulp vitality.

Eugenol: Obtained from oil of cloves, and having similar properties and uses.

Fluorides: Topical solutions, pastes, gels, toothpastes, and mouth-washes used to reduce dental decay.

Formalin: A colourless liquid with a pungent smell. A 10 per cent solution is used to fix or preserve biopsy specimens before sending them to the pathology laboratory. Formalin tablets are used to keep sterilized instruments such as reamers in a sterile state. They are placed together in tightly stoppered bottles.

Formocresol: A mixture of formalin and cresol used as an antiseptic in root-canal therapy.

Friar's balsam (compound benzoin tincture): An inhalation used for clearing nasal and sinus blockages. A dessertspoonful is added to a pint of boiling water and the vapour is inhaled. In order to prevent loss of medicated steam the patient's head and face are covered with a towel.

Glycerin: A colourless syrupy liquid which is an excellent solvent for many drugs including thymol.

Glycerin of thymol: A mild antiseptic and rubefacient mouthwash.

Hydrocortisone: A hormone obtained from the adrenal cortex. It has an anti-inflammatory action. It is used in tablets to treat aphthous ulcers, and in pastes to treat infected pulps (e.g., Ledermix).

Hydrogen peroxide: A colourless and odourless liquid available as 10, 20, and 100 volume solutions. On contact with living tissues and inflammatory products it gives off oxygen and then forms water. It deteriorates unless kept in tightly stoppered dark bottles in a cool place. The 20 volume solution is used after reaming in root-canal therapy and for bleaching blackened non-vital teeth. A dilute solution is a useful antiseptic mouthwash for the treatment of acute gingivitis.

Iodine: Blue-black prisms soluble in water, alcohol, and chloroform. It is used in solution or tincture as a mucosal antiseptic prior to inserting a needle.

Iodoform: A weak antiseptic used to eliminate infection in dry sockets and to promote healing. It is applied on gauze.

Kri liquid: A root-canal sterilizing agent.

Kri paste: A yellow root-canal antiseptic filling paste, consisting of Kri liquid and iodoform. Any excess paste forced through the root apex is resorbed.

Lignocaine hydrochloride: A very potent local anaesthetic, often used as a 2 per cent solution, e.g., Xylocaine, Xylotox. Adrenaline may be added in a proportion of 1 in 80,000 as a vasoconstrictor.

Methylpentynol (Oblivon): A hypnotic, sometimes used to premedicate nervous patients.

Nikethamide (Coramine): A liquid stimulant injected to increase the rate, and depth, of respiration. Injected when patients experience difficulty in breathing during a general anaesthetic.

Nitrous oxide: A quick acting general anaesthetic used in conjunction with oxygen. It is kept in blue coloured cylinders.

Noradrenaline: A vasoconstrictor used instead of adrenaline.

Oil of cloves: An obtundent and disinfectant. Mixed with zinc oxide it is used for linings and dressings. It has a strong taste and smell and gives rise to a burning feeling when in contact with the mucosa. The lips should be coated with petroleum jelly prior to putting clove oil mixtures into the mouth.

Paracetamol: An analgesic.

Parachlorphenol: More bactericidal but less caustic than phenol. It is used as an antiseptic during root-canal therapy.

Penicillin: A yellow antibiotic used as cones, tablets, injections, creams, and powders.

Phenol (carbolic acid): Faint pink crystals soluble in water, alcohol, and glycerin. It is very caustic so should not be allowed to contact skin. If it does so, then the area must immediately be swabbed with alcohol or glycerin, but not with water. It is very bactericidal so may be used to sterilize instruments which cannot be boiled; but all remaining phenol must be removed before using the instrument. A 5 per cent solution is occasionally used to destroy pulp remnants in root canals.

Polyantibiotic paste: A mixture of antibiotics used to sterilize root canals. It is more effective than using a single antibiotic, e.g., a mixture of penicillin, bacitracin, streptomycin, and sodium caprylate, in a silicone base.

Procaine hydrochloride: A very effective local anaesthetic. It may cause dermatitis if it comes into contact with the skin. Often used as a 2 per cent solution with the addition of 1 in 50,000 adrenaline (as a vasoconstrictor), plus sodium chloride, chlorocresol, and sodium metabisulphite, e.g., Novocain.

Sal volatile (aromatic spirit of ammonia): A stimulant used mainly for reviving patients who feel faint (syncope).

Salt water: An emetic.

Silver nitrate: Used as a 5 or 10 per cent solution or as a stick. It is caustic and astringent, acts as a bactericide, and is obtundent on exposed dentine. Seldom used now as it blackens the teeth.

Sodium chloride: Household salt. One teaspoonful in a glass of hot water is used as an antiseptic mouthwash.

Sodium hypochlorite (Dakin's Solution): A powerful antiseptic used to wash root canals after reaming. It helps to remove debris and has an antiseptic action. As Milton it is used to clean plastic dentures. A 1 per cent solution of the fluid diluted with 10 parts of water is an effective mouthwash for gingivitis.

Sodium perborate: White crystalline powder which releases oxygen on contact with moisture. A 2 per cent mouthwash is used as an oral antiseptic against Vincent's infection.

Sodium ricinoleate: A mild antiseptic incorporated into some tooth-pastes.

Tannic acid: Dilute solutions are used as astringent mouthwashes. In powder form it arrests bleeding from sockets.

Tetracyclines: A group of antibiotics with a wide range of bacteriostatic action.

Thymol: Antiseptic and obtundent. Originally used on the base of cavities prior to filling them.

Tincture of iodine: 2·5 per cent iodine and 2·5 per cent potassium iodide in 90 per cent alcohol. Used as a skin and mucosal disinfectant, and counter-irritant.

Trichloracetic acid: Colourless crystals with characteristic smell. Used as a caustic to remove infected gum flaps and to cauterize aphthous ulcers.

Whitehead's varnish: A compound paint of iodoform, benzoin, storax, balsam, and ether. Used as a varnish dressing after operations on the mouth and lips and for dry sockets.

Zinc chloride: Powerful antiseptic, astringent and caustic. It is used as a solid stick or a 10 per cent solution. Dilute solutions are used as mouthwashes. A useful obtundent for sensitive dentine.

Zinc oxide: A white powder. No taste or smell. One of the most widely used substances in dentistry. Used with eugenol as a sedative dressing in cavities and infected sockets, and for post-gingivectomy packs.

DANGEROUS DRUGS ACT

All drugs must be kept in a locked cupboard when not in use. The Dangerous Drugs Act requires strict records to be kept of all drugs coming within this category, including cocaine, morphine, and the barbiturates. Details should be recorded in a book with the following columns.

Date obtained	Supplier	Drug	Quantity obtained

This record must be retained in the practice for at least two years, and should be available for inspection when required.

These drugs can be administered by a dentist himself, or under his direct supervision and in his presence.

QUESTIONS

1. What are the uses of the following drugs or medicaments in dentistry?
   a. Ethyl chloride.
   b. Hydrogen peroxide.
   c. Vaseline.
   d. Iodine.
   e. Silver nitrate.
   f. Zinc oxide.
2. What is meant by the following properties of drugs or medicaments?
   a. Sedative.
   b. General anaesthetic.
   c. Local anaesthetic.
   d. Antiseptic.
   e. Antibiotic.
Give examples and method of use of each in relation to dentistry.
3. Describe the following drugs and their uses:
   a. Eugenol.
   b. Phenol.
   c. Absolute alcohol.
   d. Sal volatile.
4. Discuss the drugs used in dental surgery to stop bleeding.

CHAPTER XXI

ASSOCIATIONS, COURSES, AND EXAMINATIONS

ASSOCIATION OF BRITISH DENTAL SURGERY ASSISTANTS

THE major organization for dental surgery assistants, receptionists, and dental secretaries. Its aims are:—

1. To encourage the provision of facilities for practical and theoretical instruction for dental assistants in dental hospitals and colleges of further education, especially for those studying for the National Certificate. Also, to improve and standardize the training of dental assistants.

2. To assist the regular publication of articles of general interest to dental assistants and for study purposes, by means of its monthly journal. Also to form a library.

3. To assist members in such matters as employment.

4. To co-operate with the various organizations in the dental profession in order to increase the standard of dental assisting.

5. To organize meetings in all areas of the British Isles.

6. To maintain a central headquarters to which all members may apply for advice and assistance.

This Association is really a must for all dental surgery ancillary staff. Further particulars may be obtained from The Secretary, Association of British Dental Surgery Assistants, Bank Chambers, 3 Market Place, Poulton-le-Fylde, Lancs. FY6 7AX.

BRITISH ASSOCIATION FOR DENTAL AUXILIARIES

Student and qualified auxiliaries can obtain details from the Honorary Secretary, B.A.D.A., c/o London Hospital Dental School, Whitechapel, London, E.1.

BRITISH DENTAL HYGIENISTS' ASSOCIATION

Hygienists and students can join this Association by writing to the Honorary Secretary of the Association, c/o Eastman Dental Hospital, Grays Inn Road, London, W.C.1.

ROYAL SOCIETY OF HEALTH (DENTAL AND ALLIED GROUP)

The only professional organization in the United Kingdom to hold regular joint meetings for all members of the dental team, including

dentists and surgery assistants. It is therefore well worth joining.
Details may be obtained from the Secretary, Royal Society of Health,
13 Grosvenor Place, S.W.1.

NATIONAL CERTIFICATE FOR DENTAL SURGERY ASSISTANTS

This certificate is awarded by the Examining Board for Dental
Surgery Assistants. The examination is held twice yearly. There is a
written paper, practical test, oral, and ' spotter ' test. The written part
includes essays as well as a number of multiple-choice type of questions.
Before entering for the examination candidates are required to have
experience as a dental surgery assistant, or have successfully completed
a full-time course of study approved by the Examining Board. Entry
forms and past examination papers may be obtained from the Board at
Bank Chambers, 3 Market Place, Poulton-le-Fylde, Lancs.

Courses for Surgery Assistants

Many full- and part-time courses are held in dental hospitals and
technical colleges. The number of centres is continually increasing.
Full details may be obtained from the Examining Board.

DIPLOMA IN DENTAL HEALTH EDUCATION

Details of the syllabus and examination forms can be obtained from
the Examination Secretary, Royal Society of Health, 13 Grosvenor
Place, London, S.W.1.

TRAINING OF OTHER ANCILLARY PERSONNEL

Details of courses and examinations for dental auxiliaries, hygienists
and technicians may be obtained from the General Dental Council,
37 Wimpole Street, London, W.1.

HINTS FOR EXAMINATION CANDIDATES

One need hardly say that you cannot expect to get through examinations without working hard. However, this does not mean concentrated
cramming just before the examination. What is needed is steady
application throughout the full period of preparation. Textbooks alone
are not sufficient for this type of subject. Theory must be backed up by
continual practice of those techniques required of a chairside assistant.
Employers can help by giving vivas and practical tests on all aspects of
the work, including recognition of instruments. Note-taking is
absolutely indispensable. Only those with good memories know how
much they forget. Make notes of each book consulted, everything you

are told at lectures, and each new thing that you come across in the surgery. The worst ink is better than the best memory. A loose-leaf notebook is very suitable for this purpose. Thus, when you start final revision for the examination, all information will be readily on hand; even more important, it will be available for reference throughout your working life.

If possible try to attend at least a part-time course of lectures. This will enable you to learn more about your chosen subject from the lecturers, to discuss this with other students on the course, and to learn what is happening in other practices.

Work through the test questions in this book and obtain one or two sets of recent examination papers. Without consulting your notes write brief answers to the questions. Then ask your employer to go through them with you. Learn to answer only the actual question. Do not put in extraneous matter. You will gain few marks for this, and may even lose some. Answers should be written clearly, concisely, and intelligently, and the writing must be legible. When answering questions never refer to information given in a previous answer. Each must be complete in itself. Most important, before starting, carefully read any instructions given at the top of the paper. Care with all these points will pay in the long run.

Remember, '*work works*'.

EXAMPLES OF TYPES OF MULTIPLE-CHOICE QUESTIONS

1. State if the following statements are true or false:—
   a. Oxygen cylinders are black.
   b. Zinc oxide is a local anaesthetic.
   c. The heart beats 72 times a minute.
   d. The pulmonary artery contains oxygenated blood.
2. Complete the following:—
   a. Plaster is an   material.
   b. Amalgam is a   material.
   c. Codeine is an   .
   d. Lignocaine is a   .
3. Finish these sentences:—
   a. Fluothane is to a general anaesthetic as lignocaine is to a
        .
   b. Full dentures are to plaster as partials are to   .
   c. Cribs are to orthodontic appliances as lingual bars are to
        .

d. Pliers are to orthodontics as elevators are to

4. Are the following items used as stated ?
a. Post crowns to restore vital teeth.
b. Copper ring impressions for full dentures.
c. Gold inlays for fractured incisors.
d. Silver points for endodontic therapy.

GLOSSARY

Abrasion: Wearing away of surface of a material by a harder material.

Abscess: Collection of pus within a confined space.

Abutment: Terminal supporting teeth on which a bridge or saddle of a tooth-borne denture rests.

Accelerator: Chemical that speeds up a chemical reaction so that it can occur within a practical period of time.

Adhesion: Force of attraction between the surface molecules of one body, solid or liquid, and those of an adjacent one. They need not be of the same material.

Alginates: Irreversible hydrocolloids used as impression materials.

Alveolus: Portion of bone forming socket around a tooth.

Amalgamation: Reaction that occurs between mercury and amalgam alloy.

Anaesthesia: Loss of all sensations, including pain, with or without loss of consciousness.

Anaesthesia, block: Prevention of conduction along nerve-fibres by placing a chemical on the main nerve-trunk supplying fibres to the area.

Anaesthesia, general: Loss of sensation produced by putting the patient to sleep, thereby preventing reception of pain stimuli by the brain.

Anaesthesia, infiltration: Prevention of conduction by placing the chemical on the terminal nerve-fibres at, or close to, the site production of pain stimuli (e.g. at site of operation).

Anaesthesia, local: Localized loss of pain sensation produced by preventing conduction of stimuli along a nerve, by placing a chemical somewhere along its length.

Anaesthesia, topical: Loss of pain by application of anaesthetic sprays, solutions, pastes, and ointments to the surface mucosa or skin, from where they penetrate through the outer epithelium to reach the nerve-fibres.

Anaesthetics: Induce loss of sensation by local or general means.

Analgesia: Loss of pain sensation without loss of consciousness.

Analgesics: Afford relief from pain.

Annealing: Process of making a metal or alloy softer and thus easier to use. It is heated to some predetermined temperature below its melting point, maintained at that temperature for a time, and then cooled. Gold is cooled quickly, steel slowly.

Anodynes: Relieve pain by local action.

Anorexia: Lack of appetite.

Anterior: Towards the front.

Antibiotics: Chemical substance produced by micro-organisms, which are capable of destroying or inhibiting growth of other micro-organisms. Some are bactericidal (e.g. penicillin). Others are bacteriostatic (e.g. tetracyclines).

Antidotes: Substances which counteract poisons.

Antipyretics: Reduce fever or body temperature.

Antiseptics: Bacteriostatic agents which inhibit growth and action of bacteria.

Aplasia: Lack of formation of cells.

Articulating surface: Part of a bone which enters into formation of a joint.

Articulation:
1. Joint between two or more bones.
2. Forming of sounds of speech.
3. Relationship between upper and lower artificial teeth as set up in the laboratory.

Astringents: Substances which coagulate superficial cell layers to create a protective skin over the surface. This stops bleeding and acts as a barrier against invasion by bacteria and irritants. Used as mouth-washes they protect inflamed and swollen mucous membrances, and check hypersecretion. They also act as haemostats and styptics.

Atrophy: Reduced size of a tissue or organ due to a reduction in size of individual cells.

Bactericides: Substances which kill bacteria.

Bacteriostats: Substances inhibiting growth and multiplication of bacteria without actually killing them.

Balanced occlusion: Articulation of dentures such that when the teeth are brought together in any functional position, the greatest possible number of cusps are in contact and under equal pressure.

Base plate: Temporary base on which bite blocks and trial wax dentures are set up.

Bite: Relationship between upper and lower teeth or jaws.

Bridge: Prosthetic device consisting of artificial teeth suspended between abutments. It may be fixed at one or both ends, but is occasionally removable. In America partial dentures are sometimes known as ' removable bridges '.

Brittleness: Tendency to sudden fracture with slight deformation.

Buccal: Towards the cheeks.

Canine: Pointed eye tooth used for tearing food.

Carat: A measure of gold content.

Carbides: Hard compounds of metals with carbon.

Carbohydrates: Food substances which provide the body with energy, and may be converted to fat, i.e. all starches and sugars.

Carbohydrates, refined: Those which have been processed to change their consistency, colour, or taste.

Caries: Tooth decay.

Carrier: Someone who carries organisms in his body without having the disease, is incubating the disease, or is convalescing from it.

Catalyst: Material that initiates a chemical reaction.

Catarrh: Inflammation of mucous membranes, including the linings of nose and throat. May be accompanied by a discharge from the irritated tissues.

Caustics: Substances which burn or corrode organic tissue.

Cauterize: Removal of organic tissue by heat or chemicals.

Centric relation: Most retrusive, unstrained, position of the mandible.

Cervical margin: Constricted part of tooth between crown and root.

Cingulum: Ridge on the palatal aspect of maxillary anterior teeth.

Clasp: Metal attachment on a partial denture or other appliance that provides retention by gripping a tooth.

Close bite: Natural relationship of the jaws such that the space between upper and lower ridges is abnormally small.

Closed bite: Unnatural approximation of the ridges resulting from loss of natural teeth, sinking of dentures, or incorrect assessment of vertical dimension.

Cohesion: Force of attraction exerted between the atoms or molecules of substances made of similar materials.

Composite: Material composed of two or more constituents which has properties intermediate to the two portions.

Compressive strength: Stress required to rupture a material when it is pressed together.

Concave: A depression.

Condense: Compression to form the hardest possible mass.

Condyle: Smooth rounded projection of bone which forms part of a mobile joint.

Conservation: Restoration of tissue by means of fillings, inlays, and crowns.

Contact: A person who has been near to someone having a disease, and who may be carrying incubating organisms in his body. He may have to be isolated until the period of incubation is over.

Contact point or area: Part of the tooth in contact with the adjacent tooth.

Convex: A bulge.

Counter-irritant: Agents that cause surface irritation, thereby taking away attention from discomforts elsewhere.

Crown: Part of the tooth normally present in the mouth.

Crown, artificial: Means of restoring lost tooth tissue and lying mainly outside the remaining tooth structure. It takes the form of a cap made of porcelain, acrylic or metal.

Cusp: Elevation on the occlusal surface.

Dentinal tubules: Microscopic channels that extend from the pulp through the dentine.

Dentine: Hard part of tooth below enamel, which is sensitive to heat, cold and pain.

Denture: The total number of natural teeth which develop in an individual.

Denture, artificial: Artificial replacement for natural teeth.

Denture base: That part of a denture adapted to the mucous surface and which carries the artificial teeth.

Desquamation: Separation and falling off, as scales of dead surface skin and mucosa cells.

Die: Replica of a tooth on which an indirect inlay or crown is made.

Direct technique: The shaping of a wax pattern on the prepared tooth itself.

Disinfectants: Agents which destroy living organisms by bactericidal, germicidal, or fungicidal means.

Distal: Away from the midline.

Elasticity: Characteristic of a material which enables it to recover its initial shape and size after deformation.

Emetics: Substances which induce vomiting.

Enamel: Hard cover on crown.

Face bow: Device to record the relationship of maxillae to glenoid fossae, of ears, to enable models to be correctly orientated on the articulator.

Facet: Small flat articulating surface of bone.

Fever: Rise in temperature with accompanying signs and symptoms.

Fissure: Depression between cusps of tooth, or in bone.

Food: Any solid or liquid which can be used by the body for its living functions (growth, repair, reproduction, production of energy).

Foramen: Hole in bone, for passage of vessels and nerves.

Fossa: Shallow depression on any surface.

Frankfurt plane: Plane passing through the lowest part of the orbit and the highest part of the tragus of the ear. It is horizontal when the head is in a normal upright position.

Gangrene: Necrosis plus infection by putrefactive (pus-forming) micro-organisms, which thrive upon dead cells.

Gingival (cervical): In the region of gingivae.

Haemostats: Mechanical or chemical agents that arrest bleeding.

Hardness: Measure of the resistance to indentation of the material by either a hardened steel ball or a diamond point.

Heat treatment: Process of heating an alloy to a selected temperature below its melting point, and then cooling at some predetermined rate so as to obtain specially required properties.

Hygroscopic: Tendency to absorb water from the air.

Hyperplasia: Increased size due to an increased number of cells, not to their enlargement.

Hyperpyrexia: Rise of body temperature to more than 104 °F.

Hypertrophy: Increase in size of a tissue or organ due to enlargement of the individual cells.

Hypnotics: Drugs which in normal doses induce sleep similar to natural sleep, helping patients to have a good night's rest before a dental operation. Small doses act as sedatives, e.g. barbiturates, chloral.

Incisal edge: Cutting or tearing part of incisors and canines.

Incisors: Anterior teeth which incise or cut food.

Incubation period: Interval between the invasion by infecting organisms and the first signs and symptoms of the disease.

Indirect technique: The shaping of a wax pattern on a model (die) of the prepared tooth.

Infusions: Preparations formed by pouring boiling water on to a substance and then straining it, e.g. tea.

Inlay: A solid pre-formed filling cemented into a suitably prepared cavity.

Interdental space: Triangular area between two teeth below contact point. It is usually filled with gum tissue (interdental papilla).

Interstitial or proximal surface: Surface facing the next tooth; therefore mesial or distal.

Intravenous: Into a vein.

Labial: Towards the lips.

Lingual: Towards the tongue.

Malaise: General feeling of being unwell or run down.

Malocclusion: A condition in which the cusps of upper and lower teeth do not meet in the normal way.

Mandibular: In the lower jaw.

Marginal ridge: Mesial or distal elevations on the occlusal surface.

Maxillary: In the upper jaw.

Mesial: Towards the midline.

Model: A replica typically made of plaster that is used primarily for study purposes.

Molar: Posterior grinding tooth.

Mould: A hollow cavity into which melted material is introduced to form an object.

Mouth protector: An appliance made to fit over the teeth of the maxillary arch to protect them from injury.

Naso-tragal line: Imaginary line joining the lower border of the ala of the nose and the upper border of the tragus of the ear. The occlusal plane is approximately parallel to this line.

Necrosis: Death of cells and tissues.

Nutrition: Process of assimilation of food, i.e. its use by the body.

Obtundents: Drugs which dull sensations such as pain, including that from exposed dentine, e.g. oil of cloves, zinc chloride.

Occlusal rest: Projection from a denture which rests on some part of the occlusal surface of a natural tooth to prevent the denture from sinking down on to the mucosa.

Occlusal surface: Cusped chewing portions of molars and premolars, which occlude with the teeth of the opposing jaw.

Occlusion: Meeting of upper and lower natural or artificial teeth or bite blocks.

Onlay: Means of raising the height of occlusal surface. It is often used in the treatment of temporomandibular joint disfunctions.
   1. By modification of an inlay so that the bulk of the material is external to the tooth rather than filling a cavity in it.
   2. By modification of a denture so that the acrylic teeth rest on the natural teeth.

Open bite: Condition in which a group of natural teeth are unable to meet when the remainder are in occulsion. The opening may be anterior, posterior, unilateral, or bilateral.

Oral cleanliness: State of the mouth as seen at examination.

Oral hygiene: Sum of all the measures practised by dentist and patient to achieve a satisfactory state of oral cleanliness, and through this to attain and maintain maximum oral and dental health.

Orthodontics: The study of cause, prevention and treatment of irregularities of shape of the jaws, and position of teeth.

Overbite: Downward projection of the upper incisor tips below the level of the lower incisor tips.

Overjet: Forward projection of the upper incisor tips in front of the lower incisors.

Palatal: Towards the palate.

Papule: Nodular elevation of skin, seen with certain rashes.

Paraesthesia: Increased and abnormal sensations.

Partial denture: A prosthetic device containing artificial teeth supported on a framework and attached to remaining natural teeth by means of clasps.

Peripheral seal: Seal which should exist around the outer edge of a full denture to hold it in place. Its existence depends on the correct extension, shape and thickness of the denture margins. In the upper jaw a posterior seal is produced by the yielding tissues at the junction of hard and soft palates.

Photophobia: Discomfort with light.

Plastic: Material capable of being moulded into a new shape under the influence of heat and pressure.

Pontic: Part of a bridge holding artificial teeth.

Posterior: Towards the back.

Prodromal: Early symptoms of a disease, prior to main clinical manifestations.

Prophylaxis: Any method used to prevent disease, e.g. vaccination, fluoridation, toothbrushing.

Prosthesis: Appliance which replaces lost or congenitally missing tissue, anywhere in the body.

Prosthesis, dental: Although by definition this should include fillings and crowns, the term is normally reserved for such appliances as artificial dentures, bridges, obturators, and surgical prostheses.

Prosthetics: Restoration by full or partial dentures. Bridges are sometimes regarded as fixed prostheses.

Pulpectomy: Complete removal of the pulp.

Pulpotomy: Partial removal of the pulp.

Pustule: Small swelling on the skin surface filled with pus.

Pyrexia: Raised body temperature.

Quadrant: One half of the maxilla or mandible, i.e. a quarter of the total jaws.

Raised bite: Jaw relationship in which the jaws are unduly separated by dentures on which the teeth have been elevated by some chairside or laboratory error.

Relief chamber: Depression in the fitting surface of an upper denture to prevent rocking over a relatively hard area, or to reduce pressure on a tender or sensitive part of the ridge.

Relining: Re-adaptation of fitting surface of a denture by adding a layer of fresh material.

Resorption: Physiological removal of bone by special cells (osteoclasts) after tooth extraction, leading to a gradual reduction in size of the bony ridge.

Retention: Resistance against any force that tends to dislodge a denture.

Root: That part of the tooth which is normally fixed in bone and thus not seen.

Rubefacients: Substances that increase blood-flow to the skin in the region to which they are applied, providing warmth and some degree of counter-irritation, e.g. hot-water bottle, oil of wintergreen.

Saddle: Part of denture resting on or covering the alveolar region.

Sedatives: Drugs which calm nervousness or fear by partial depression of the central nervous system. Small doses act as tranquillizers and large ones as hypnotics, e.g. alcohol (ethyl alcohol), phenobarbitone.

Sialogogues: Substances which increase the flow of saliva, e.g. lemon juice and clove oil.

Sinus: Hollow cavity within bone.

Styloid process: Sharp downward projection of bone for attachment to muscles and ligaments.

Styptics: Drugs which are applied locally to control bleeding, e.g. alum, tannic acid.

Survey line: Line of maximum bulbosity of a tooth in relation to the path of insertion of a denture.

Sutures:
1. Immovable joints between bones.
2. Stitches used in surgery.

Syrups: Substances dissolved in a solution of sucrose in water.

Tempering: Heat process to alter the hardness of a metal.

Thermoplastic: Reversible property of becoming softer on heating and harder on cooling.

Tinctures: Solutions of drugs in alcohol.

Tranquillizers: Drugs that promote a sense of well-being or calmness, with no clouding of consciousness or impaired intellect, e.g. short-acting barbiturates such as phenobarbitone.

Traumatic occlusion:
1. In the case of natural teeth, traumatic occlusion is one where tooth cusps of one jaw bite abnormally against one or more cusps of the occluding teeth, with resultant damage to their periodontal membranes and sockets.
2. With artificial dentures, it is due to a raised bite or to poor articulation preventing natural movements of the mandible. Injury occurs to mucosa, periodontal membrane, and sockets of nearby natural teeth.

Trituration: Process of mixing mercury with amalgam alloy.

Varnish: Resin surface coating formed by evaporation of a solvent.

Vesicle: Blister of skin or mucosa, e.g. in chickenpox and shingles.

Vibrating line: Line of junction between the movable tissues of the soft palate and the static hard palate. It is the correct position for the posterior margin of an upper denture.

Vitamins: Chemical substances essential to normal health that occur naturally in many foodstuffs, e.g. ascorbic acid, riboflavine.

INDEX

Gingivectomy, 167
 instruments for, 113, 123, 168
Gingivitis, (Fig. 32) 64, 148
 acute ulcerative(Vincent's), 84, 88,
  167, 169, 219
 chronic marginal, 84, 85
 marginal, 166–7
 of pregnancy, 85
Gingivoplasty, 167, 169
Glands,
 alimentary, 9
 facial, 55
 lymph, 54–6, 67, 68, 84, 85, 86, 212
 lymph, groups of, 54–6
 parotid, 37, 45, 51, 54, 55, 213
 salivary, 9, 14, 24, 36, 37, 45, 50, 55
 sublingual, 36, 46, 50, 55
 submandibular, 36, 46, 50, 54–6, 67,
  213
Glass-ionomer (ASPA) cement, 133,
 137, 149
Gloves, 69
 sterile, 160
Gold crown, 132–3, 142, 151–2
 inlay, 132–3, 142, 151–2
Guild of Barber Surgeons, 1
Guild of Surgeons, 1
Gutta percha, 140, 216
 sterilization of, 93

Haemophilia, 65, 69–70
Haemorrhage (see Bleeding)
Haemostats (see also Bleeding), 28, 166,
 215, 216
Halitosis, 85
Handbook for National Health Service
 General Dental Practitioners, 4
Handpieces, 113, 124
Hare lip, 57
Health Educator, 5
Health, training courses for, 219
Heart, (Fig. 6) 15
 coronary circulation, 20, 21
 disease, 23
 failure, 69, 189–90
 structure, (Fig. 6) 18
 valves, (Figs. 6, 7) 20–1
Heat, in sterilization, 92, 94
Hepatitis, acute infective, 90, 91, 94
 serum, 183
Herpetic stomatitis, 86, 169
Hertwig's sheath, 58
Hiccough, 17
History of dentistry in the United
 Kingdom, 1–6, 185
Hormones, 22
Hospital Dental Service, 1, 3
Hospital, Royal Dental of London, 1
Hospitalization for haemophilia, 69–70
 for shock, 73
Hydrocol, 138

Hygiene, oral, 76, 81, 82, 83, 85, 175,
 178–80
 personal, 103, 160
Hygienist, 5
 duties of, 5
 training courses for, 221
Hygienists' Association, British Dental,
 221
Hyoid bone, (Fig. 15) 40, 42, 44–5
Hyperaemia, 73, 79, 133
Hyperplasia, 71–2, 167
Hyperpnoea, 17
Hypersensitivity, 96–7
Hypertrophy, 71
Hypocalcification, 58
Hypoplasia, 58

Immunity, natural and acquired, 91,
 95–6
Impacted teeth, 60, 163–4
Impression compounds and techniques,
 137–43, 157–9
 copper ring, 139, 151, 152
 for crown, 139, 152–4
 dentures, 139, 157–9
 materials, 137–43
Incisors, (Figs. 12, 24, 37, Table II) 35,
 52, 59, 64, 76, 109
Infection, 23, 58, 65
 control of, 22, 90, 166
 droplet, 17, 91, 212, 213
 reactions to, 68
 resistance against, 68, 91
 spread of, 36, 67, 90–1
 symptoms of, 68
Inflammation, 66–8, 72, 90
 acute, (Fig. 28) 66
  sequelae of, (Fig. 28) 67–8
  symptoms of, 66
 chronic, 68
 protection, 66–7
 repair, 67–8
Influenza, 90
Injections (see also Anaesthesia), 165,
 183–5
 when to avoid, 70
Injuries to teeth, traumatic, 85, 156
 205
Inlay, 6, 112, 135
 gold, 132, 142, 151–2
 porcelain, 132, 137, 151–3
 wax, blue, 142, 151
Instruments (see also Equipment), care
 of, (Fig. 34) 102, 105–6
 functions of, 112
 illustrations of, 114–24
 sterilization of, 92, 94, 102, 160–1,
 216, 218
Intestines, (Fig. 8) 15, 24, 26
Iodine, 93, 217
Irradiation, 92